Pregnant at 16

Lori Ghiata Bowser

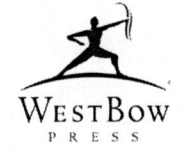

WestBow
PRESS

Copyright © 2010 Lori Ghiata Bowser

All rights reserved. No part of this book may be used or reproduced by any means, graphic, electronic, or mechanical, including photocopying, recording, taping or by any information storage retrieval system without the written permission of the publisher except in the case of brief quotations embodied in critical articles and reviews.

WestBow Press books may be ordered through booksellers or by contacting:

WestBow Press
A Division of Thomas Nelson
1663 Liberty Drive
Bloomington, IN 47403
www.westbowpress.com
1-(866) 928-1240

Because of the dynamic nature of the Internet, any Web addresses or links contained in this book may have changed since publication and may no longer be valid. The views expressed in this work are solely those of the author and do not necessarily reflect the views of the publisher, and the publisher hereby disclaims any responsibility for them.

ISBN: 978-1-4497-0293-9 (sc)
ISBN: 978-1-4497-0294-6 (hc)
ISBN: 978-1-4497-0292-2 (e)

Library of Congress Control Number: 2010928612

Printed in the United States of America

WestBow Press rev. date:5/12/10

"The mercy of the Lord is from everlasting to everlasting."
Psalm 103: 17

For our first precious grandchild,
Lindsey Brooke Bowser
(Dan and Erin's princess)

DEDICATION

*"For You formed my inward parts;
You covered me in my mother's womb.
I will praise you, for I am fearfully and wonderfully made.
Marvelous are Your works.
And, that my soul knows very well.
Psalm 139: 13-14*

    Lovingly and respectfully, I dedicate this book to those remarkably courageous, unwed, pregnant teenage girls who have chosen to do the right and honorable thing by giving life even in the midst of anxiety, turmoil, and negative whispers from onlookers.

    In case you've never heard these words, *"Good for you!"*

"God will bless you beyond your dreams for your unselfish decision."

CONTENTS

PART 1: WHO IS SHE?   1

CHAPTER 1   DO YOU KNOW HER?   3

CHAPTER 2   KEEPING SECRETS: THE SKELETON IN MY CLOSET   21

PART 2: CHALLENGES   69

CHAPTER 3   ADOLESCENCE   71
CHAPTER 4   PEER PRESSURE   78
CHAPTER 5   TEEN PREGNANCY   87
CHAPTER 6   TEEN MOTHERHOOD   104
CHAPTER 7   TELLING MY KIDS   119
CHAPTER 8   TELLING MY ADULT FRIENDS   125

PART 3: TAKE A CHANCE ON A TEENAGER   131

CHAPTER 9   BEFRIENDING TEENAGERS   133
CHAPTER 10   BEFRIENDING PREGNANT TEENAGERS   148

PART 4: GOD'S BLESSING   151

CHAPTER 11   BLESSINGS BEYOND MY DREAMS   153

ACKNOWLEDGMENTS

*"Open your mouth for the speechless,
In the cause of all who are appointed to die."
Proverbs 31: 8*

It has been my honor throughout the writing of my story to acknowledge genuine admiration for my parents, Donald and Thais Ghiata. Their unfailing and unconditional love that has been repeatedly demonstrated toward me has given me an awesome lead to follow and bright stars to reach for.

Though I relentlessly challenged my parents' patience in my adolescence, they faced those challenges head-on with dignity, grace, and Godly perseverance.

Thank you for loving me, Mom and Dad.

If my children and grandchildren have even half the loving feelings for me as I do for you, then my soul will be satisfied.

Most assuredly, you are my heroes!

Deep gratitude is extended to my husband, Joe, for causing me to believe that my dream of reaching out to others with my story can be a dream come true.

Thank you for understanding my passion for speaking up for those who cannot speak for themselves/the unborn, and my unwavering pledge to be their very loud voice.

Joe's soft reminders of God's *still, small voice* deepened my passion to challenge others to show compassion toward teenage unwed mothers.

His gentle nudges encouraged me to throw caution to the wind and follow my dreams wherever they may lead.

My story has a happy ending.

Or, should I say it *ends with a beginning* - of happiness, wherewithal, and fortitude.

Ultimately, it is because of the birth and life of my son, Danny that I was inspired to author a work intended to encourage teenagers, teenage girls in particular, to follow their dreams, reach for the stars, and never ever give up or give in.

Danny, you are not only my inspiration, but you are my undeserved blessing.

I am so proud of the fine man you have become, and it is my honor to be your mom.

Thank God for your mark on my life - a *mark* I am proud to show off.

Danny, Shannon, and Shelby, I am so thankful for the love the Lord has shown to me through *each* of you.

You *all* have blessed me beyond my dreams.

This story is for the three of you, your children, and your children's children.

Though this is a story you have *heard* time and time again, it is a story that comes from my heart and deep within my soul.

Now that it is in written form it is a story that you can *share* time and time again in detail with loved ones for generations to come.

To God be the glory!

FOREWORD

"You shall not follow a crowd to do evil..."
Exodus 23: 2

The title pretty much gives it away, doesn't it? Here I sit, thirty-five years later, at long last loosening the constricting noose from my burdened neck, releasing the agonizing clamp from my tightly sealed lips, and baring my soul while resting in the hope that this writing will open eyes, expand minds, and enlarge hearts.

I am finally ready and more than willing to share my story about what it was like to find out at only sixteen too-young years of age that I was pregnant.

Finally!

Yep, you're actually hearing it from the horse's mouth this time, not from one of those onlookers who just take Danny's age and subtracts it from my own and wonders - making what he or she considers to be educated guesses at my history.

Ah, what an oppressive weight is being lifted from deep within my soul as I write this.

To get this cumbersome load off my weary shoulders, and to finally speak openly about my teenage pregnancy, rather than keeping it all bottled up inside me, is not only a gargantuan step and leap of faith for me, but it is very freeing as well.

The year was 1974.

It was the tail-end of the *hippie, free love* and *peace* era.

We had just pulled out of the Vietnam War one year earlier.

The Beatles had already convinced us that *"love was all we needed."*

The Civil Rights Movement was still in its infancy.

By this time the Women's Lib Movement had gained enormous strength and stressed that women had *"come a long way, baby"*.

And, legalized abortion was brand spanking new.

Being an unwed pregnant teenager at that time was possibly an even heavier weight to carry on one's shoulders as compared with present day.

In fact, I'll go out on a limb and say that indeed it was a heavier load to carry than now-a-days.

Consider this. Today you get the news that the girl next door, or the cheerleader in high school, or even the preacher's daughter, gets pregnant. Perhaps this news is initially surprising to you, but it's just that - a mere *surprise*.

Quickly, you and others may accept the fact that this young lady is expecting a baby, and perhaps even embrace the anticipation and excitement of a new life in progress.

On the other hand, if the young girl chooses to terminate the pregnancy, you and others (depending on whether you are pro-life or pro-choice) may think little or nothing of this fact, since abortion is unfortunately so commonplace now.

Let me remind you, however, that in the early 1970s legalized abortion was brand spanking new.

Furthermore, an unwed mother at that time was condemned by most if she carried the baby to full-term *and* condemned by most if she had an abortion.

You could say it was a lose/lose situation.

It was almost certain that she would be convicted, being made to feel she had committed a crime. Perhaps even the unpardonable sin.

Either way, the shock and embarrassment of teenage pregnancy was a heavy cross to bear.

It's not that it was a rare event for teenagers to have premarital sex at that time. It wasn't that at all.

Remember. *Free love.*

But even though the love was free, it was nonetheless kept more *hush-hush* back then.

Yeah. *Secret free love.*

Girls had exceptionally good secret-keeping skills.

Boys - not so much!

They preferred to bring all this secret free love stuff out in the open, sharing it quite proudly with each other and with pretty much everyone else.

But, that hasn't really changed much over time.

Clearly, boys have a genuine fondness for spreading the news regarding their own sexual encounters – particularly, the ones that are simply made up in their own minds.

Aside from boys' unrelenting desires to verbalize their sexual interactions with girls, back in those days, we avoided openly discussing even the subject of *marital* sex, let alone *pre-marital* sex.

It has long been my impression that perhaps many adults in that period of time felt that if it wasn't talked about, it wasn't happening - an *out of sight/out of mind* kind of mindset.

Adolescents' curiosity about and interest in sex, however, is an age old occurrence adults must deal with in a straightforward manner.

Straightforwardness did not appear to be an attribute held by the majority of parents of teenagers in the 1960s and 1970s.

My sweet parents were the exception to that rule.

They were considerably straightforward, as a matter of fact. My problem was - well … me.

Rest assured, I do not now nor did I then dance to the beat of a different drum, but I am incredibly hard-headed.

My mom likes to say that I get that from my dad.

Likewise, my dad likes to say that I get that from my mom.

Who knows?

In any case, I am ever-learning to soften my hard head.

I think I am gaining more success at this personal project with each passing year.

I think!

But every now and then, and sometimes more *now* than *then*, my head is like concrete.

Let's just say I am a work in progress.

God is not finished with me yet.

If you are my age or older (I was born in 1958), you likely have a pretty clear picture of what a pregnant teenager might have had to endure during the 1970s.

If you are younger than me, particularly if you were born in the 1970's or later, the picture might be a little fuzzy.

Please allow my story to create for you a more vivid representation.

Note:

This is *my* story.

Mine!

Though it may bear striking similarities to other stories of this nature, this particular story is wholly and completely *mine*.

Therefore, my prayer is that it will not be torn apart by anyone reading anymore into it other than what is simply stated from my heart.

Please keep this in mind as I bear my soul.

PART ONE

WHO IS SHE?

CHAPTER ONE
DO YOU KNOW HER?

*"Before I formed you in the womb,
I knew you."
Jeremiah 1: 5*

She's probably a friend, a neighbor, or even a loved one. No matter what your present age, you more than likely know of an unmarried young lady who has either had a child out of wedlock or had an abortion.

Perhaps you know one or more of each.

Perhaps that someone is yourself.

Typically, in this day and age, when folks hear of either a young mother having had a child out of wedlock, or a young lady having had an abortion, it is not a shock to one's system.

Generally, no one is particularly astounded by news of this nature.

Presumably, this is due to the fact that teenage pregnancies and pregnancies outside of marriage have become quite commonplace today.

The commonality of it all seems to have caused a widespread numbing of our minds, our hearts, and without a doubt - our morals.

It has been my experience that minds without morals and heartlessness were not quite so prevalent in the early 1970s as compared with present day.

Though hippies and other teens in the 1970s were singing their songs about peace and free love, I would venture to say that they held themselves to a somewhat higher moral standard when compared to many of today's teenagers, and adults for that matter.

Let me also suggest that the greater portion of teenagers in the 1970s demonstrated considerable evidence of respect for authority figures - including their parents, teachers, and law enforcement officers.

For example, in the 1970s there was not a need for student resource officers that are found in most public schools today. The teachers, the principals, and other adult personnel were quite capable of disciplining the students as needed without outside reinforcement.

And, we were more intolerant of foul language at that time.

Think about it - if you were alive back then.

Television programs and radio stations were *censored* on those matters.

Many teenagers now have no idea what we're talking about when we mention *censorship*. Just ask them.

I'm going to take even one step further out on that limb at the risk of making myself sound like an *old timer*.

Well, maybe a few steps.

If one could take a class of high school students from the 1970s and intermingle them in the same room with a class of today's high school students, the 1970s kids would stand out like handfuls of sore thumbs, not because of the way they would be dressed, but because of the way they would present themselves.

I'm quite certain that even the thugs and hippies from the 1970s would appear strangely meek when standing side by side with the thugs and gang members in today's classrooms and school hallways.

I have formulated my certitude regarding this matter from having walked those hallways personally at two different eras of my life - during the 1970s as a student, and recently as a health occupations teacher at a local high school.

The striking similarity between the 1970s kids and today's kids however, is that within the heart every teenager - the real *heart of the matter* - there lies a soul just begging to be loved and understood.

My mom frequently remarks, *"They say there's nothing new under the sun."*

She's right.

There's not.

But, it is quite possible that those same *old* things can decline with time.

The rapid decline of moral standards in our society, for example, is a crying shame, but not shocking.

Why should we be shocked?

Society is not taking care of business. Society is not practicing what it preaches.

Kids learn quite well by example, whether that example is or is not appropriate.

Furthermore, at that time in history (the 1970s), when a teenager was a willing participant in anything considered to be wrong, especially when that *something* might result in pregnancy, adults could be quite vicious in word and in deed.

Arguably, adults were not the only creatures capable of cruel behaviors.

The adolescent's peers could be quite vicious as well.

As a matter of fact, peers generally don't hold anything back. They just let the cruel comments fly.

In the 1970s, if you had an abortion, nobody knew it. It was mega hush-hush.

So, typically those girls didn't have to deal with negative peer pressure, and neither did the boys who participated in the impregnating of the young ladies.

Nope.

The only ones who were made to deal with ruthless, heartless, and brutal comments of others were the girls who decided that two wrongs do not make a right and kept their babies, or at least carried them to full term and then gave them up for adoption; unless –

Unless they married the father of the baby, which happened fairly routinely because the parents of the young teenage couple convinced them that they had to get married.

Had to get married.

Now, there's a phrase that's outdated. And anyone who has ever been married knows that marriage does not solve anything.

It certainly does not solve problems.

Rather, marriage can be a too well-known creator of problems.

And in the same manner that people are able after all this time to take Danny's age and subtract it from mine and figure out that, yep, he was born to me while I was a teenager - did those parents not think that the community would surely come to the conclusion that the teenagers' wedding bore a striking resemblance to a shotgun wedding?

It doesn't take a math wizard to take the date of the wedding and the child's birth date and subtract one from the other and come up with –

You've got it.

Less than 9 months.

Even so, the *had-to* marriages apparently seemed to those intimately involved in the situation to be the quick fix, the perfect answer, the pardon for the sin.

On the flip side and not surprisingly, those marriages typically ended up in divorce court.

Still do.

Evidently, the parents who made their children get married hadn't considered the fact that the marriage might not last for all eternity.

By no means, is this a newsflash.

Young people are still being forcefully encouraged to get married if a pregnancy occurs out of wedlock.

Allow me to recount a fairly recent true story that creeps into my memory with relative frequency.

It's my case in point, if you will.

Several years ago, a teenage couple I knew very well found themselves faced with their own pregnancy out of wedlock. When each of the parents of this young couple found out about this circumstance, or predicament, as I believe they considered this situation to be, the young couple was not only encouraged to make things *right* by getting married, but also to confess publicly in their home church, in front of the congregation on a Sunday morning, their inappropriate behaviors and the resulting pregnancy.

What?

I don't recall other *sinners* being convinced to endure humiliation in front of the church body in this manner.

Here are my problems –

No! Here are my genuine, heart-felt concerns with all that:

- I am convinced that the couple would not have stood in front of the congregation confessing their sins if they had not been *caught* by the unexpected pregnancy and persuasively convinced by authority figures of the need

- to verbally admit their *guilt* to the entire church body on that very difficult Sunday morning.
- Marriage doesn't make an unplanned, out-of-wedlock pregnancy *right*. The sex out of wedlock is still wrong, marriage ceremony or no marriage ceremony following the realization of the child in the womb.
- The marriage ultimately ended in divorce. So, as the story goes, instead of one wrong as it regards this young couple's indiscretions, they now have two:
    1. the sex outside of marriage; and,
    2. the divorce.

It is not necessary to confess our sins to anyone except God, Himself.

Most importantly, the Bible tells us that when we make these confessions, *"He is faithful and just to forgive us our sins, and to cleanse us from all unrighteousness." - 1 John 1: 9*

Let me just add that when I heard of this young couple's pressure into publicly confessing in front of the entire church body, my heart went out to them.

I mean, if confessing in this manner was really necessary, where were all the other *sinners*?

The others surely did not make their *sinful voices* heard.

Not *that* Sunday morning.

Not *any* Sunday morning!

The young man and young woman in this couple were and still are very sweet people with hearts full of love for the Lord.

So, they made a mistake.

An error in judgment.

Don't we all?

And don't we do it with relative frequency?

I do.

I try not to, but we are all born with a sinful nature.

And Satan continues to work so relentlessly at petitioning us to join his cause.

He is especially working hard on the born again Christians, because those who do not claim to know Jesus are already in Satan's Army.

He's already won that battle.

I, on the other hand, am in the Lord's Army. I have decided to follow Jesus. And I will fight the battle against Satan until I take my last breath.

I am choosing not to give in to my sinful nature, though I admit I sometimes have a failure rate of which I am less than proud.

Much less.

Thank God that I am able to be *cleansed from all unrighteousness* when I confess my sins to Him. Take that, Satan!

There's an old saying that suggests time changes everything. I disagree.

I do believe that time has the ability to dim memories sometimes, and to make past wounds less painful.

Nonetheless, the memories and wounds are still there, or at least the scars remain.

Scars are reminders that never go away. They can only fade over time.

In fact, it has also been my experience that there are quite a large number of things that time itself cannot erase.

Time cannot erase reality.

And it is impossible for time to erase history.

Historically speaking, then, something that is not likely to change with time is the fact that many folks of all ages continue to talk perversely about the unwed teenagers that carry their precious babies to full term.

Talk about perverse!

Carrying a baby to full term rather than choosing abortion is anything but perverse.

Instead, it is the very right and very moral choice.

Unfortunately though, history has also shown me that the majority of those folks that speak perversely about unwed teenage mothers are the same folks that speak passionately about the teenagers who have abortions - the ones who put an end to the lives of their babies.

Yes, you read that right!

I could have chosen to be more politically correct and stated, "the ones who *terminate their pregnancies.*" But, that just seems too generic a translation for an act that is specific.

Specifically, when someone chooses to have an abortion, the reason is to remove the human fetus so that its development is arrested and the baby dies.

Moreover, I've never been a fan of *political correctness*. Rather, I prefer to just tell it like it is. *I call 'em as I see 'em.*

I can do that, you see, because I happen to be *one of 'em*. Most assuredly, I am not one to pull punches or to sugar-coat wrong-doings. Not even my own. Not anymore anyways.

Some might argue that sometimes a pregnancy is terminated, or a precious baby's life is ended, to protect the health of the mother.

Here's a reality check for you. Rarely, is that the case. At least not when compared with the number of abortions being performed for the sake of convenience.

I challenge you to do your own deep, investigative studying on that precise subject.

You'll see for yourself that my statement is not merely a *theory*.

I have had the opportunity in my line of work (I am a registered nurse of seventeen years) to discuss this issue with many medical providers who are *pro-choice*, and what I have learned from their

Pregnant at 16

input is that they are of the mind-set that the mother's *health is protected* by having an abortion if she is not emotionally or mentally prepared to have a child.

So, when you are conducting your own investigative study and reading your statistics, keep that tidbit of information in mind.

I have also had the *heart-wrenching* experience in my career to hear parents persuading their teenage daughters to have abortions, even when that is not the choice the teenager really wants to make.

I have heard these parents telling their sweet daughters, *"It's the right thing to do";* and, *"This is the best decision for you and your baby";* and even, *"What kind of life would the baby have if it was born while you are so young?"*

Right to have an abortion? No!

Best decision to have an abortion? No!

What kind of life? How about this: an opportunity to experience a wonderful, fun-filled life just like any other child born to anybody else.

To sum it all up, the choice for life is the best choice.

No!

It is the *only* choice.

Indeed, there should be no other choice/no other option. However, there are many options once the child is born.

For instance, adoption is an amazingly wonderful alternative to eliminating a precious life by enduring a gruesome and heartbreaking abortion procedure, let alone the mental torment and anguish experienced by the aborted child's mother either immediately or sometime further down the road.

Historically speaking again, *abortion* has been defined as a miscarriage or an untimely, inopportune, or premature birth.

In the present day, however, the term *abortion* is most often recognized as the removal of a fetus by choice simply because the mother feels the arrival of a living baby at this time in her life is untimely or inopportune, and perhaps she feels she simply cannot emotionally handle the energy required to provide for the child.

This is not new news!

At this present time in history, the majority of abortions are not miscarriages.

Rather, they are the taking of a life by choice.

Even if I had chosen to travel down the abortion road myself in 1974 (which I did not), I am certain that I would still be matter-of-fact in defining abortion and the *wrongness* of it all. It's what one might call a *no-brainer*.

In fact, I'll be the first to admit when I make a mistake, or to admit guilt regarding my own sins.

To be honest, I haven't always been of that particular frame of mind.

Through the years though, I've been made keenly aware that I'm not the only one who makes mistakes. Far from it, in fact. And it is this realization that has made it much easier for me to finally become forthcoming and verbally acknowledge to others my own self-inflicted and heart-wrenching mental torment caused by my own mistakes, and how I overcame the guilt and shame (which is actually still a work in progress, by the way).

Thank God, I am not alone.

Thank God!

And I believe, from the bottom of my heart, that others who have made some of the same mistakes I've made are glad to hear from someone who has *been there* like myself.

And, this is the motivation for writing my story - to help others realize:

- that they are not alone;
- that there really is a bright light at the end of every tunnel; and,

- that there is a beautiful rainbow at the end of every *storm* in your life.

God has been with me through all of my *storms,* and Danny was the *bright light* that God blessed me with at the end of my *tunnel* as well as the *beautiful rainbow* after my *storm.*

Finally – at long last – I can accept and admit my own mistakes, and thus forgive myself rather than carrying my shame and guilt to my grave, which is the direction in which I was erroneously heading for the past thirty-five years.

One of my past sins – one of too many, I might add – was having sex out of wedlock.

There I go again – calling a spade a spade.

My resource for defining sins?

The Bible.

As you are reading this, you may be thinking I'm a little old-fashioned - maybe even a little prehistoric.

You are wrong.

Dead wrong!

I am very aware of and in tune with how things have changed over the years.

But, I also believe that over the years our minds have become more and more corrupted by our sinful nature.

The Bible is not old-fashioned, nor is it prehistoric.

Its truths just happen to remain unchanged, making the Bible a timeless work of non-fiction.

Doubting Thomas?

The following are some Scripture references regarding sexual relationships:

- *"Avoid sexual immorality." – 1 Thessalonians 4: 3-7*

- *"Since there is so much immorality, each man should have his own wife, and each woman her own husband." – 1 Corinthians 7: 1-5*
- *"If they cannot control themselves, they should marry, for it is better to marry than to burn with passion." – 1 Corinthians 7: 8-11*
- *"The body is not meant for sexual immorality. Flee from sexual immorality." – 1 Corinthians 6: 9-20*

Since the definition of the word *immoral* might be a little confusing to some folks, let's allow dictionary.com to define that for us:

"Violating moral principles; not conforming to the patterns of conduct usually accepted or established as consistent with principles of personal and social ethics."

And in case some folks may be puzzled regarding the use of the term *ethics*, again, according to dictionary.com, *ethics* refers to:

"A system of moral principles; that branch of philosophy dealing with values relating to human conduct, with respect to the rightness and wrongness of certain actions and to the goodness and badness of the motives, and ends of such actions."

To clarify even further then, *my* personal understanding of *sexual immorality* is this:

"Sexual immorality is a behavior or pattern of behaviors that do not conform to accepted rules of society, but that also are not consistent with God's perfect plan for a relationship between a man and a woman.

Indeed, sexual immorality does not at all measure up to God's expectations for emotional and physical behaviors exhibited by humanity – creatures of His perfect design.

To be sexually immoral is to purposefully choose to disobey God's rules in the game of life."

Having made reference to God's word, permit me to repeat *with emphasis* that my sex out of wedlock was a sin!

Yes, I am pointing an unyielding finger at myself.

On the other hand, I have yet another uncompromising finger, again pointing at myself but more precisely at my heart, reminding me that my resulting pregnancy was not a sin.

Rather, it was a *cause and effect* kind of happening. I *happened* to get pregnant because I *happened* to have sex. The *effect* was the pregnancy that was *caused* by the sex.

So let us be ever mindful that pregnancy is never a sin. Conversely, destroying a pregnancy is most assuredly a sinful act. Sure, I became pregnant because of the sex, but the pregnancy resulted in my undeserved blessing.

Danny.

When I asked God for His forgiveness for my immoral behaviors, He did so much more than just forgive me.

He turned my shame into honor.

Yes!

He honored me for confessing my sin to Him and, it is my honor to be Danny's mom. My blessed honor!

My dad was the first one to explain to me that two wrongs do not make a right. I already committed one wrong, and was not willing to complicate matters by committing yet another one.

Not a chance!

A decision for abortion would have been just one wrong sitting smack dab on top of the other.

The lives of the unborn are very important to God; and, the Bible tells us that there is a penalty to be paid for harming a fetus.

Still doubting?

Consider these Scripture references.

- *"If there is serious injury (to the unborn child), you are to take life for life, eye for eye, tooth for tooth, hand for hand, foot for foot, burn for burn, wound for wound, bruise for bruise." – Exodus 21: 22-25*

- *"For you created my innermost being; you knit me together in my mother's womb. I praise you because I am fearfully and wonderfully made; your works are wonderful, I know that full well. My frame was not hidden from you when I was made in the secret place. When I was woven together in the depths of the earth, your eyes saw my unformed body. All the days ordained for me were written in your book before one of them came to be."* – Psalm 139: 13-16

God's word is crystal clear on the abortion issue.

And just as clearly, abortion causes much more than merely a *serious injury* to the life of a fetus.

Given my own teenage history, I expected it might be somewhat tricky to instruct my children in the importance of saving sex until marriage.

I figured they would always respond to my *lessons learned* speeches with, *"Hey, you did it, mom."*

Surely, that thought may have raced through their minds at times.

At other times, the thought may have just stood in one place in their one-track minds.

But, at least they were respectful enough to me to refrain from verbalizing that thought to my face.

And, even if they did choose to express their feelings to my face, or even behind my back – no matter … my memory is dim.

Regarding my own parents, they are God-fearing, loving, born-again Christians for whom I have the utmost respect and admiration.

In fact, they continue to be my role models, daily, and I love them dearly.

My mom is innately wise and compassionate, with a gentleness that has calmed every storm I have ever faced. Every one!

She has taught me so much, both in word and by example.

My dad is absolutely the most biblically wise man I have ever met in my life, and his love is beyond compare.

Lovingly, I joke that they should have named a book of the Bible after him – *The Gospel According to Don*.

He probably wishes that I hadn't put that in writing here, because he is humble as well.

My dad is not a preacher, but he practices what he preaches.

I just wish I would have been more receptive to his *sermons* as a youngster.

Being a parent and grandparent myself now, I can only imagine that my teenage pregnancy must have initially tormented my parents' souls.

Further, hear this and remember it well - though my parents hated the *sin*, they loved the *sinner*.

They loved *me!*

They loved me in the same manner that my God, my Father in Heaven loves me.

Despite my sometimes disrespectful, sinful behaviors, they embraced me with their love.

My parents have always supported me emotionally.

That emotional support during my teen pregnancy was and still is so appreciated.

All unwed, pregnant teenagers desperately need love and emotional support.

And I remain in awe of my parents' ability to have so effectively and lovingly met my needs during my unexpected pregnancy.

In fact, they are my example of how I want to pay it forward, so to speak, and provide emotional support for pregnant teens today.

My parents provided me with financial support as well, but they had to dig deep in their pockets, because neither I nor my precious baby, Danny were covered under any insurance plan.

None!

So, my pregnancy was not an easy experience for my mom and dad either.

Nope.

It was costly.

Indeed, a high price was paid for my poor choices, in more ways than one. Admittedly, I made some very unwise investment decisions. Talk about the high cost of living!

I learned some valuable lessons from my experiences, however.

After I turned my life back over to Jesus, allowing Him to guide my life decisions, I gained the knowledge that Jesus loves me even with all my shortcomings.

I was given considerable insight into His mercy, forgiveness, and grace.

Get this: He even gave me a *refund* on my indiscretions.

Yes, he paid me back - with interest.

Praise God for my undeserved blessing - Danny!

That, my friend, was an excellent investment.

My decision to put everything I had within my soul into carrying through with my pregnancy, and then raising Danny to the very best of my ability, has proven over and over again to be an investment that consistently reaps benefits beyond whatever I could have hoped or dreamed.

Make no mistake, God's refund and reward to me was not due to my own errors in judgment; but, I am convinced it was due to my genuine request for His forgiveness for my mistake as well as my decision to follow through with the pregnancy, and to raise and nurture Danny to understand the teachings of the Lord Jesus Christ, and to encourage him to cultivate a close personal relationship himself with Jesus.

Until now, I have kept my story a secret, at least from anyone who is not either family or a very close friend with whom I felt my secret was very safe - safe from the minds of those who might whisper negativities, point shameful fingers, or pierce my heart with fiery darts.

Shame on me!

Shame on me for not sharing this story years ago.

Looking back, I think that secrecy was part of Satan's handiwork.

I have since decided that I cannot and will not let Satan win.

Not only do I want to tell my story, but I'd like to shine a very bright light on it. Everything out in the open. No more secrets.

My intentions regarding this endeavor are many and diverse.

Initially, my objective was merely to open the eyes of those who choose to close not only their eyes, but also their minds and their hearts to those unwed pregnant teenagers and teenage mothers who so desperately need to be accepted, understood, and loved.

I have since decided, however, that there are a few other avenues worthy of being considered.

In particular, I will address the seemingly insurmountable, timeless challenges facing pregnant teenagers and teenage mothers.

I have chosen to make myself transparent.

Transparency of self is a road I have not traveled until recently.

Previously, I steered clear of this bumpy road because of the risks involved in traveling through unknown territory.

Currently, I am choosing to give myself the green light to travel down Transparency Road, allowing others to view my past as well as to see into the very depths of my soul.

This forth-coming of self carries with it the potential of being an invitation for harsh criticism from people from all walks of life.

On the flip side, there is the possibility that my initial objective may be met and eyes will be opened, minds will be expanded, and hearts will be enlarged.

This is a risk I am more than willing to take in an effort to allow outsiders to get a glimpse into the mind, and a window into the soul of at least one who has *been there*.

If you have been there, or if you are there now, my prayer is that my story will be a blessing to you and inspire you to be all that God wants you to be.

You are His daughter, and He loves you with all His heart.

There is no greater love than His.

Remember the song you may have learned in Sunday School as a small child – "*This Little Light of Mine?*"

Just as the song reminds you, don't hide your *light* for Jesus under a bushel, or anywhere else for that matter.

Rather, *"Let your light so shine before men, that they may see your good works and glorify your Father in Heaven." – Matthew 5: 16.*

Let it shine!

Let it shine!

Let it shine!

CHAPTER TWO
KEEPING SECRETS: THE SKELETON IN MY CLOSET

*"Deliver those who are drawn toward death,
And hold back those stumbling to the slaughter."
Proverbs 24: 11*

A very kind lady once told me that everyone has a skeleton in his or her closet.

When those words first fell upon my ears, I wasn't quite sure about their meaning.

After her brief explanation, however, I realized that I had several of those scandalous bones locked up in my very own closet.

Still do!

There is one skeleton still hidden, in particular.

Until now, I have hidden that skeleton key very carefully, and have been vigilant about guarding that key with my very soul.

Though I've let a few curious folks take a peek into my deep, dark closet, it has only been a brief peek at best.

I've never really been too crazy about the idea of exposing my skeleton to the outside world. After all, outsiders can be awfully critical regarding a skeleton such as mine.

It can be a *cold, cold* world out there. And, I have always wanted to protect my skeleton from the outside elements.

In addition to the *cold*, I didn't think it wise to allow my skeleton, or myself for that matter, to be exposed to the *heat* either.

So, I chose to safeguard my skeleton from the *elements* by keeping it securely locked in my closet. And I was the only one allowed to carry the key.

You see, though those close to me knew of my skeleton, they were *warned* that it was never, ever allowed to leave the safety of my closet without my permission.

The *heat* being transmitted from others toward my direction over the years has been a little too hot for me to handle at times.

It might appear to an outsider looking in that I deal with criticism quite well.

But, nope!

Never been a fan of criticism.

Throughout this manuscript, you will see evidence of my skeleton key turning – slowly, but with determination.

But, before I make that first purposeful turn, allow me to express what I believe caused me to put my skeleton in the closet in the first place.

I am convinced that we begin to collect our skeletons during adolescence. I collected the majority of mine during that time.

Why adolescence? More than likely, it's due to enormous peer pressure. You know - the pressure to be like everyone else in your age category.

I don't think we ever outgrow peer pressure. Rather, we just learn to handle the pressure with a little more maturity and grace as we age, or at least I'd like to think that's the case.

Adolescence is a time of uncertainty, to say the least. Teenagers are desperately and constantly trying to figure out who they are and where they fit in.

Sometimes the teenager's quest for fitting in can lead to some reckless behaviors.

Characteristically, the teen does not necessarily think hasty behaviors are particularly reckless at the time.

It is a well-known fact that teens have an *"it'll never happen to me"* attitude. Typically, they fail to see beyond the here and now.

Furthermore, teenagers have an incredibly omnipresent need to be accepted by their peers.

Peer acceptance and not looking toward the future can lead to errors in judgment. Very often, those poor judgment calls translate into an ever-present *keepsake* for the remainder of our lives.

Some of those *keepsakes* are right out in the open, and some we keep locked up tight.

I will get to my very own skeleton momentarily, but first allow me to give my own definition of just a select few of the teenage peer groups.

Peers fall into a variety of categories or *crowds*, if you will.

Let's face it, no matter what our age, we all want to be a part of the *in* crowd.

As adolescents, we are bombarded with crowds from which to choose.

The following is an abbreviated adolescent crowd list.

- the SMART kids
- the NOT-SO-SMART kids
- the ATHLETIC kids
- the MUSICAL kids
- the INTROVERTED/SHY kids
- the EXTROVERTED/CONFIDENT kids

- the CHRISTIAN kids
- the STREET-SMART kids

Typically, kids are a combination of a few categories.

When kids are describing other kids however, they generally place an individual into only one category, that category being the one that most effectively describes the personality of an individual.

Even thirty-plus years after high school, I can name names of which of my former classmates fell under which category.

They were all stand-outs.

Whatever your age, you can probably do the same thing.

I recognize that we all change as the years pass; and, most of us have hopefully aged gracefully, having transformed ourselves into more than just the *stand-out* that we were in high school.

SMART KIDS

In high school, I would have loved to have been classified as a *smart kid*. How awesome it would have been to be one of those students who knew the answers to every one of the teacher's questions!

To hear a piece of information once or twice and have it stick in my brain forever, being able to retrieve it at a moment's notice. That would have rocked my world.

Unfortunately, my world was not yet set in a rocking motion at that time.

In fact, it was peculiarly motionless.

No, I did not possess the genius gene.

But I did inherit its distant cousin, the cleverness gene.

I'm not quite sure which of my ancestors passed this gene on to me, but I was a master at having it work to my advantage.

I am convinced that many other teenagers, former and present, have been blessed with that gene as well.

The cleverness gene causes us to figure out brilliant ways in which to make our not-so-brilliant minds work in our favor.

For example, I consistently aced my high school science tests one year. This was not because I was a science geek. Rather, I owe it to my science teacher's method of preparing the students for his tests.

Simply stated, my teacher was a creature of habit. Well, either that or he was just lazy.

Back in those days there was no such thing as teacher accountability.

My science teacher just used the same boring method of test preparation for each and every test.

Without fail, you could count on the fact that his tests would have thirty questions.

Prior to test day, he would verbally quiz us with the very same questions that would appear on the upcoming test.

In fact, he would go around the room asking those questions in order. He would ask student number one question number one, student number two question number two, student number three question number three, and so on.

There were thirty-two students in our class.

Incorporating my cleverness gene, I made sure that on *verbal quiz day* I always sat in seat number thirty-one or thirty-two.

Conversely, the really *smart kids* always sat in seats one, two, and three.

Are you following this yet?

You've got it!

By sitting in seat number thirty-one or thirty-two, it was only necessary for me to simply memorize the answers given by the *smart kid* occupying seat number one or two in the classroom.

In so doing, and by the time the teacher got around to verbally quizzing me, I too was able to give the correct answers to the test questions by merely regurgitating the *smart kids'* answers.

Clever?

You betcha!

At least for that year in my life, I considered it even a splendidly ingenious plan.

Note that I did not declare that it was a *genius* plan, but rather an *ingenious* plan.

There's a difference, you know.

Yep! Here comes the language lesson from one who formerly considered herself to be a *not-so-smart kid*. According to <u>Webster's Handy College Dictionary</u>, to be a *genius* is to have *"exceptional mental and creative power"*; but, to be *ingenious* is to show *"cleverness in contrivance or construction."*

To contrive and/or construct – that was me, baby. It was a *glitch in my system*. Hey! It worked for me.

That is, until I got much older, thirty-two years old to be exact, when I entered Nursing School. Then, I had to incorporate a different plan of attack, though far from being original.

The plan?

Simply study.

Nothing more.

Nothing less.

So, to any current students who may be examining this text, don't be misguided. My *ingenious* plan was anything but.

Instead, it caused me to have to go *back to the basics* in college, having to study probably twice as hard - or more - as those who were prudent enough to study in high school.

NOT-SO-SMART KIDS

Nobody aspires to claim the title of the *not-so-smart kid*. Unfortunately, however, there are some poor souls who might just as well have this title plastered across their foreheads.

Worse yet, these kids are likely the ones you may recall seeing walking down the school corridors, totally oblivious that some bully has plastered across their backside the word *stupid* or, the infamous words *kick me*.

They're the ones unfortunately destined to be on the receiving end of bullies remarking, *"Oh yeah, you know him, he's the one with the dumbfounded look on his face all the time."* Or, *"When they were passing out brains, that chick just got in the wrong line"*. And let's not disregard the ever-popular slam, *"He's so dumb, his dog teaches him tricks"*.

I remember quite well those kids on the receiving end of those comments.

Target practice for bullies is unmistakably their fate.

Why is it that these poor kids stand out like a painfully sore thumb?

And, why are we able to so easily spot them - a mile away, as they say?

I think it's the insecurity factor that gives them away. They're generally the ones who are uncomfortable with eye contact. They don't perform well in conversations either.

And, since they aren't even fortunate enough to have inherited the cleverness gene, they have no self-defense mechanism.

I'm sure you have heard it said that it's better to be quiet and have people think you're stupid, than to open your mouth and remove all doubt.

Well, maybe that's a form of passive self-defense.

Given that fact, maybe the *not-so-smart kids* are verging on brilliant after all.

Seriously, what gives us the authority to deem someone *not-so-smart* anyway?

I can think of a multitude of *smart kids* I went to school with who still don't know enough to come in out of the rain.

And I can name a few folks even now who are book smart, but stand out in the *thunderstorms of life* without possession of a *common sense umbrella*.

Moreover, what is the definition of *smart*?

Do you really know?

Are you sure?

Go ahead. Look it up in the dictionary, but only after you've made an educated guess in your own mind of its meaning.

Now that you've done that, did you determine that maybe you are *not so smart* after all?

And, *who* defines *smart*?

The teachers?

Don't be so quick to jump on that train of thought.

Though I am familiar with many teachers who seem to *have it all together* and appear to be a *book of knowledge*, I can effortlessly see in my mind's eye just as many that would cause me to run to the front of the line in order to passionately debate the theory that all teachers are intelligent enough to define *smart*.

So, you kids out there who are tempted to believe you're *not so smart* - don't be too quick to wear that crown either.

In fact, don't accept that title at all. Not now, and not ever!

Everyone is different. Everyone is an individual.

Don't ever let anyone tell you that you're not smart enough to do something/anything.

Yes, you are!

Perhaps you might have to work a little harder at accomplishing your goals or dreams than another person, but that doesn't mean that you can't do it, or that you can't do it better than everyone else, or that you can't see your dreams come true.

Yes, you can!

Dream big.

Reach for the stars.

Your dreams as well as the stars really are within your reach. As a matter of fact, you may not have to reach as far as those bullies who give you such a hard time.

Hey! It's quite likely that the bullies are bullying you just as a cover-up for their own *not-so-smartness*.

ATHLETIC KIDS

Sometimes those bullies or *not-so-smart kids* appear in the form of an athlete.

Note to parents of athletes: In case you are feeling the heat of defensiveness creeping into your thought processes ... I said, "*sometimes.*"

Everyone seems to envy the *athletic kid*, don't they?

If the athlete is of the male persuasion, he has no problem attracting females.

If he's the athletic star, all the girls want to be his little starlet.

And, if he happens to be a rather large jock, no one is going to bother or pester him.

Clearly, if another student is enough of a half-wit to choose to annoy the monstrous athlete or to make fun of him in any way, the half-wit better be regularly watching over his shoulder due to the ever-so-obvious fact that the heavy-duty athlete could and would likely pulverize the half-wit with the slightest of effort.

If the athlete is, on the other hand, of the female persuasion, she is likely quite popular as well. She doesn't have any trouble getting guys to call her for a date, and her peers often consider her their role model.

Back when I was in high school, we didn't have very many female athletes.

The one and only reason for this was because we were made to believe that females just didn't do that sort of thing. Apparently, being athletic was unbecoming and not feminine.

So, we didn't have a girls' basketball team, or a girls' softball team; but, we did have a co-ed cross country team. But, I'm sorry to say only one girl was *manly* enough to go out for the cross country team.

Things were just different back then.

We did have cheerleaders. But, even they were not the real athletic type cheerleaders compared with the cheerleaders that we have now.

They didn't storm the ball field or the gym floor with gymnastic-style back flips and acrobatics.

Rather, they *graced* the fields and floors of sporting events with their precious demeanor, cute little miniskirts, tight sweaters, and saddle oxford shoes while chanting the infamous, *"Go team go."*

No, the cheerleaders of my day were not athletic enough to wear even athletic type shoes.

Their job was this: Be cute while cheering for the boys.

I am quite aware that cheerleaders today are entirely athletic. And, I'm delighted that schools now offer girls' softball, basketball, tennis and soccer, just to name a few sports available to young ladies.

You go, girls!

But in my high school days, many young ladies were quite content to simply look cute on the gym floor or on the football field, while cheering for the boys.

My mom says I've always *cheered for the boys.*

But, that's another story.

Nonetheless, I tried out for the cheerleading squad a few times. No success - well, at least no success in achieving a place on the squad.

On the flip side, I was successful at making people laugh. And then, cry. Or, maybe they were crying from laughing so hard. Quite likely. Picture this …

I was quite a bit taller than most of the other cheerleader wannabes, while being skinny and scrawny at the same time.

It was because of my tiny build that I earned the position at the top of the cheerleaders' pyramid.

Did these girls not know that being tall, skinny, and scrawny also makes one extremely and inevitably awkward? That was one tough lesson these girls learned by experience.

I already knew that I was awkward, but I was just too shy to say anything.

Bad combination. Though our pyramid lacked precision by any stretch of the imagination, I am sure the bird's eye view from the gym bleachers was a sight to behold.

Looking back, I have no doubt that I would have laughed out loud had I been a spectator myself that day.

In fact, I'm cracking up at the picture in my mind's eye now.

After all, I did look pretty silly when I quickly lost my balance (not really certain whether I even had any balance in the first place) and fell off the top of the cheerleaders' pyramid.

If camcorders had been available back then, our stunt may have been seriously considered for airing on one of those funniest video television programs.

I landed hard on my back on the equally hard gymnasium floor.

Immediately following that rough landing, I landed on my back again - at the emergency department.

I didn't endure any permanent injury.

If anything it just hurt my pride, and only for a negligible time.

Maybe, just maybe, that's why I didn't make the squad?

I'm not skinny and scrawny anymore, but I am still at times likened to a bull in a china shop.

Let's face it. Whether male or female, it's not really a problem or concern if the athlete is not academically gifted. It should be, but in many cases it's not. We all know that stand-out athletes stand a very good chance of getting into the best colleges, often with a full scholarship, or at least a partial scholarship.

They can be dead-ringers for *not-so-smart kids*, but many school officials just don't seem to care ... as long as they can *play ball*.

I have a vivid recollection of one particularly *athletic* kid from my high school days.

Moose.

I think every high school has one - a *Moose*, that is.

Our *Moose* was comparable to the *Moose* that you read about in the comic books. He was a very distinct character. He was as gentle and sweet as one can imagine. But, on the *bright* side of life, his personal light was a bit dim.

But, what an awesome football player! What an impressive athlete!

What an animal!

Thus, the fitting nickname.

He was so unlike me!

You guessed it. I didn't inherit the athletic gene either.

I was, beyond the shadow of a doubt, among the most athletically-challenged.

In order to give you a small sampling of my athletic disabilities, allow me to recount for you my painfully pathetic high school basketball story.

We were in gym class learning the ins and outs of playing the game of basketball.

My gym teacher informed me that I would be playing *defense*.

What?

I was under the impression that the entire game was a defensive game.

And *offense*? New word. What in the name of heaven was that?

No, I didn't know the difference between defense and offense.

And I sure didn't know that I would have to switch back and forth between the two *'fenses*. Sheesh! Too complicated!

Evidently, my gym teacher made the unmistakable discovery of my defense/offense discombobulation much faster than - well, much faster than I did.

So, being the sympathetic and kind lady that she was, she patiently but matter-of-factly went to great lengths to teach me the monumental differences between playing defensively and offensively; and, even went so far as to tell me specifically where to stand on the court.

This was all so confusing to me!

Remember, I told you I was athletically challenged.

We've already had this discussion.

Anyway, as I recall (and I recall very clearly by the way, because embarrassing moments have a way digging a very deep groove in your brain, you know), I was to stand directly under the net (just *one* net) and defend my team by making sure that the players on the other team did not get the ball into that *one* particular basket.

Not wanting to disappoint my teacher, and desperately wanting to let her know that not only had I listened intently to her explicit directions, but that I was going to be the queen of my defensive basketball kingdom - I planted my feet firmly under that *one* basket, and *only* that *one* basket - for quite some time!

I thought, *"Well, this is boring."*

Yep, even when all (*all!*) of the other players ran to the basket at the other end of the court, I was cemented to my defensive part of the basketball court.

I did not follow their lead.

I had never been accused of being a follower, and I wasn't going to start then. No way! Not me, buddy. My job was to protect that one basket, and only that one basket.

I ... was the basketball *"goalie."*

Needless to say, the sweet, kind gym teacher that I had known and loved so well suddenly became harsh and merciless.

Had I done something wrong?

I was just following directions, and doing a darn good job at it too.

Well, she just blew me away by enlarging the molehill to mountainous proportions. And I was at the mountain's peak. All because I followed her instructions to the letter.

Go figure!

No wonder I still don't like basketball.

Dumb game! Just pick a basket. Any basket.

For all of you basketball fans out there, don't take *offense* or *defense* or ... whatever!

So far, the waters were not filling my gene pool.

MUSICAL KIDS

I began to think that maybe, just maybe, my gene pool was just patiently waiting to be filled with the gift of natural musical talent.

Consider this. *Musical* kids can be pretty cool. And, who doesn't want to be cool?

Singing is cool.

But, although I have as long as I can remember considered myself to be the *star in my car*, singing is most assuredly not a gift with which I have been blessed.

Clearly, it is not a gift that anyone would care to have me share with them.

You know this too well if you have experienced the misfortune of standing next to me while I sing my ever-lovin' heart out with every hymn on Sunday mornings.

Hey! Is that why I'm always sitting by different people in church? I could have sworn I always sat in the same pew.

Instruments like the flute, violin, or guitar - to name a few - just really weren't my cup of tea either.

But, hey - I have long fingers. On many occasions, in fact, little old ladies would come up to me and take my hand while remarking on my lovely *piano fingers*.

That was it! Of course! I would try my hands, or my *piano fingers*, at becoming *musical* by learning to play the piano.

I tried.

I failed.

I gave up when it became frightfully apparent to me how difficult it is to be a *natural talent*.

Before making that bleak discovery however, I talked my parents into purchasing a piano for me. After all, my best friend, Cindy had a piano and her mom gave piano lessons.

D-uh! Another no-brainer. Buy the piano. Take lessons from Cindy's mom. And, voila! Pianist extraordinaire!

Not!

My poor mom. She should've practiced dentistry, because persuading me to practice the piano was like extracting wisdom teeth, only worse.

I mean, why should a *natural* talent like myself be forced to practice?

I absolutely dreaded going into the family room downstairs to practice for thirty long, tortuous minutes.

This was not at all going according to my plan.

This called for *Plan B*: Take advantage of mom's hearing disability (oh, what a character I was), and just practice two or three songs that I could already play really well.

I played them over and over and over again.

Sorry, mom!

I thought I really pulled the wool over her eyes (or, *ears* in this case).

I was wrong. She's not easily fooled. Neither was my piano teacher.

Thus, the lessons didn't last for any extended period of time.

And, what was all this talk about people playing the piano *by ear*?

I tried that too.

I think my ears must have been out of tune. And try as I might, my tuning capabilities were *zip, zero, zilch.*

Well, when you fall off the horse, you're supposed to get right back on, correct?

I didn't immediately remount the horse, but fifteen years later I decided to make an attempt at climbing back on that piano bench, and to place my piano fingers appropriately on the white and black keys of our beautiful Grinnell Brothers piano.

This time I was somewhat more successful, and I did practice.

After all, I was the one paying for the lessons this time.

Having a little more faith in my piano fingers, I accepted a substitute pianist position one Sunday, and only one Sunday, at church.

You'll understand the reasoning behind my one-time claim to fame momentarily.

My acceptance of this position was not without a little reluctance, but I accepted it nonetheless. After all, we went to a small country church, and it's important that everyone share their talents for the betterment and fulfillment of the church body. And, how bad could it be?

Pretty bad, actually.

Read on!

I had all my ducks in a row. I like them that way!

I practiced and practiced, and practiced some more. Yes - just the same hymns over and over again.

I informed Connie, the organist, which songs we would be playing together that Sunday.

I even took it one step further, and practiced with her on a couple of occasions the week prior to my first (and only) professional appearance.

To cover all bases, I also took it upon myself to inform the church secretary which songs to list in the church bulletin for that particular Sunday.

My *ducks* were lined up perfectly.

Or, so I thought.

Oops! I forgot to tell the song leader.

Failure to do so, led to quite a catastrophic incident.

Sure, the hilarity of it all makes for quite an entertaining story at parties - now. But at the time, dreadful humiliation filled my entire being.

God's way of incorporating humbleness into my soul?

Possibly.

Ron, our song leader, announced the first song to the congregation.

Then, he took what I considered to be an incredibly long pause, while the church members patiently held open their hymn books in preparation to sing praises to our Lord and King.

Meanwhile, I was thinking: *"What is his problem? He's not new to the game of song leadership! What's the hold-up? Why doesn't he start singing?"*

As my frustration was causing me to consider rolling my eyes and twiddling my thumbs, Ron turned to me and whispered, *"Start playing the introduction."*

I thought …

"The what?"

Oh, what I would give to have a picture showing the bewilderment in Ron's face (as evidenced by his unusually perplexing facial contortions - which included wide eyes, goofy-looking eyebrows, and bizarre deformations of his lips) when I whispered back, *"I don't know how to do that"* and, *"You just start singing and I'll jump right in"*.

Well, he just turned those bewildered tables back onto me with even wider eyes, his lower jaw now hanging down onto his chest, and arms partially outstretched, palms upward.

You get the picture.

I think he was more than just a little upset.

In a louder whisper now, and mouth wide open, he slowly and deliberately uttered words that in my wildest dreams I did not expect to hear.

As a matter of fact, I couldn't believe my ears when he confided, *"I don't know this song."*

Oooh, no! Holy Moley!

This was no wild dream, my friend. This was most assuredly a *nightmare.*

Long story short - I just started playing, and he *tried* to jump in.

My recollection of the events following our brief intermission in the church service is only as clear as mud. I'm guessing that some of the folks in the congregation must have been familiar with my choice of hymns, and temporarily played the role of self-appointed song leaders themselves by breaking out in song for the moment, and as needed.

I believe the mortification of it all has resulted in yet another dim memory for me.

You know, like one of those brain-things where you cannot for the life of you remember a catastrophic event.

Interestingly, Ron must have experienced the same brain-thing as I, because he doesn't remember the event at all.

I wonder why they never asked me substitute for the regular pianist again?

You know that horse that's always waiting to be remounted? I did it again. Just one more time.

I attempted piano lessons again just a few years back. They didn't last long. I was catching on o.k., but when you get to my age, there are just too many other things demanding our immediate attention.

So, not unlike countless potential pianists - I find myself sitting on my beloved piano bench, 40 years later, wishing I had paid more attention in piano class - the first time!

I applaud, in standing ovation style, the *musical kids*.

INTROVERTED / SHY KIDS

Still desperately seeking to *find myself*, or my place in my teenage world of confusion, I had no intention of filling my gene pool with anything remotely resembling introversion.

Or, maybe because I was so concerned with my own thoughts about *who* I was and *where* I fit in, I *was* introverted?

Who knows!

It certainly would not have been my top choice, if given a choice, to be an introverted kid, because typically teenagers avoid the introverted kids like the plague.

That is, unless they are introverted themselves.

When that's the case, the introverts tend to find each other like peanut butter finds jelly.

By themselves, they can be quite boring. But, put them together and they blend quite well, and can be quite interesting in their own nontraditional way.

It makes no difference that they are distinctively different from each other. They're okay with that because they know that they are vastly different from, and don't fit in with, the majority.

And, it is by this means that they bond together or *blend* so well.

It is not a difficult task to spot the introverts, because despite their differences from everyone else as well as each other, they still stand under the same introverted umbrella.

Some might refer to these kids as nerds or geeks.

Who wants that title?

And yes, even nerds and geeks are quite different from one another, even though they stand dreadfully close under that umbrella.

The nerds are quite often slouched over and may even look downtrodden; whereas, the geeks generally stand a bit taller.

The nerd might be wearing hand-me-clothes; whereas, the geek's choice of clothing for the day may include a long black overcoat worn so that others cannot see the clothing beneath.

The nerd may be sporting a haircut given by mom or dad; whereas, the geek has cut his own hair, styled it in a strange way, and dyed it jet black (to match the overcoat).

The nerd's presence may be unseen and unheard; whereas, the geek makes certain that everyone sees and hears him.

The list goes on and on.

But, they do have common ground.

That foundation, sadly, is the obvious lack of certain social graces.

This deficiency in social graciousness commonly translates into the introverts being relentlessly teased and mocked regarding their deviation from the norm.

Adolescents can be so cruel to others in their age group just because they're different in one way or another.

And whether nerd or geek, the insecurities of these kids are worn visibly on their shirt sleeves.

I recollect with relative ease, and quite well in fact, the awkwardness demonstrated by those considered *nerds* or *geeks* from my *personal* aimless driftings along my *own* high school hallways.

And the cruelty demonstrated to these kids by the other students hasn't really changed over time either.

I know this because I have seen it with my own eyes and heard it with my own ears.

Recently!

A few years back, I taught health occupations courses at a local high school for four years.

On a daily basis, it was made quite apparent to me that many teenagers still feel the need to humiliate and torment the introverts relentlessly.

My heart goes out to these kids who are mocked and persecuted.

Who knows what their home life is like?

Who knows what goes on behind closed doors?

EXTROVERTED / CONFIDENT KIDS

The doors to the extroverted kids' homes are likely a little sturdier, a little more desirable, and a little more open.

And, more than likely these kids have a more traditional, typical home life as compared with the introvert.

It is reasonable to think that the extrovert's personality quite possibly arises from the fact that his/her parents have greater communication with their children as compared to the *possible* dysfunctionality of the introvert's family.

My personal favorite illustration of functional communication is D.E.A.L. time. It works like a charm! At least, most of the time.

What makes it exceptionally charming from *this mom's* standpoint is that typically, kids are *oblivious* to this M.O. (method of operation).

And quite possibly, *oblivion* may be one of the greatest resources in unconventional parenting.

Mull over this one for awhile. You know how sometimes it's just hard to get your kids, especially your teenagers (who already know everything, so they don't need to discuss daily life issues or happenings with their mom or dad), to really open up and have a conversation with you? When you find yourself up against *that* brick wall, try DEALing.

Instead of bugging the living daylights out of your child by saying, "*Sit down, and let's talk*" (they hate that - they always assume they're in trouble), D.E.A.L.

Drop Everything And Listen.

Yes, stop dead in your tracks.

Whatever you are in the middle of can wait.

Yes, it can!

It can even wait until tomorrow, if need be, or longer.

Struggling with parenting schemes and designs, can be a losing battle at times. But there is not much that is more important than taking the necessary time to really listen to what your child has to say.

Genuine attention is the universal key that unlocks so many doors into your child's existence. When this key is turned, you will learn so much. Likewise, you will have the door wide open to teach your child so much.

Go ahead. Try it. You might like it.

In all probability, the extrovert's family has a similar M.O.

Let us also consider the possibility that the extrovert may very well come from a family of affluence.

Characteristically, this would allow the extrovert to have not only more opportunities than the introvert because he/she may exhibit more of an air of self-confidence, but it would also grant him/her certain advantages that the introvert would never in a million years expect to experience.

Examples of such advantages may include things like a salon haircut vs. the home grown haircut that the introvert might be forced to sport; or, trendy, stylish clothing vs. bargain basement clothing or hand-me-downs found the in the introvert's closet.

Like it or not, these things are important to teenagers. Very important!

Within the teenage society, there is a clear distinction between those who *have* and those who *have not*.

And, it has been my observation that, often (not always, but often), those who *have* frequently seem also to reside on Snob Hill.

In other words, these particular extroverted snobs seem to have the idea that they deserve nothing less than to have everything they hope for and dream of to become a reality; whereas, the introverts seem content just to hold on to their dreams, and keep dreaming.

They expect nothing; and are therefore, never disappointed.

To be fair, not all extroverts are residents of the Snob Hill neighborhood.

Just as often, there are the extroverts who are apparently just born with brains, or beauty, or personality-plus, or incredible talent. Perhaps they are even blessed in all of those areas.

Hey, it could be that they are even genuinely gracious and kindhearted toward those less fortunate than themselves.

My hope and prayer is that there are more of these graciously kindhearted kids than I realize.

I had a friend like that.

Her name was Anna Beth.

She did not come from a family of affluence, and she did not reside on Snob Hill. She was just genuinely a nice girl. She was one of my Christian friends. In fact, she was my favorite Christian friend during my teen years.

One of the sweetest things I will forever remember about Anna Beth is that when I got pregnant at sixteen years old, she wrote me the most heart-felt, loving letter and told me that she loved me and was there for me to meet any need I might have.

What a friend! What an example of Christ-likeness!

CHRISTIAN KIDS

Just like Anna Beth, most (not all, but most) of the Christian kids are generally nice to everybody. Or, at least they should be.

They are the ones you can trust with your life. In fact, they hold the key to life eternal.

I was a *Christian kid*, but not as much of a *Christian kid* as I should have been. In other words, I was not anywhere near being all that the Lord wanted me to be. Of that, I am certain.

Unquestionably, it was not my custom to visibly demonstrate or verbally reveal my Christianity on a routine basis. I regret that this must have disappointed and saddened my Savior during my younger teenage years.

My reluctance to share the gospel of Jesus Christ with my friends, and my indifference toward attending youth group activities surely must have grieved my parents as well. Nonetheless, they persevered in teaching me the things of the Lord. And I know that I was present in their daily thoughts and prayers.

There is a Scripture that says, *"Train up a child in the way he should go, and when he is old, he will not depart from it"*. – Proverbs 22: 6

Well, I am older now. Much older. And, I've not departed from *the way I should go*.

How's that for evidence of truth in scripture?

Granted, when I was much younger – specifically, a teenager – I had become fairly proficient at departing from my parents' training. I was quite skillful at *jumping the track* so to speak, certain that making my own tracks was the superior choice for myself.

Now that I am much older and at least to some extent wiser, I wish I could *back-track*, having discovered during my fifty-two years that departing from my parents' training was something much *less* than wise and much *more* than inferior.

If you are a teenager reading this now, please think twice or even three or more times before *jumping tracks* like I did.

Back-tracking in life is simply not an option. It is entirely an impossibility.

Watch out for yourself. Be wary of anything that appears to go against what God's word inspires you to do. Be cautious and look both ways before *crossing the tracks*. Stay focused enough to remain on the *right track*. Trust me – you'll thank yourself later.

Although I knew when I was just a child what I also know now as an older-than-middle-aged adult, that Jesus laid down His life for me on the cross at Calvary, I just didn't take the time to really consider the magnitude of Jesus' love for me when I was journeying through the awkwardness and selfishness of my own adolescence.

As is the case with the majority of teenagers at any given time or place in history, I was more concerned with considering my own special place in this world, desperately wanting to fit in somewhere - anywhere!

And, if luck would come my way, maybe I could earn one of the *"stand out"* titles that everyone would forever recollect from high school.

Like my peers, I longed to be accepted - to be *somebody* - not just another face in the crowd, not just another photograph in the yearbook, and not just another clone of *teendom*.

Furthermore, rather than immersing myself in the fellowship of teenagers who held the same beliefs in Jesus that I did, I chose to saturate my soul with the brotherhood (and sisterhood) of non-believers.

Why?

Why do teenagers make many of the decisions they do?

Who knows?

I didn't go out of my way to get involved in the youth group at church, or even to participate in student Bible studies at school. Well, once in a while I did. But had I opted to do so more often, perhaps the direction in my teenage world would have changed its course as a result of the forces of *positive* outside influence.

I knew deep in my heart that I loved the Lord, and wanted to serve Him, but at that time I was tremendously shy and insecure, and just wasn't the *voice* that I should have been.

Yeah, I know. Those of you who are reading this and know me too well, but didn't know me as a teenager, are likely a little flabbergasted at the *shy* piece of information, and are probably thinking, *"What?" "Shy?"* And, *"Sure! Whatever, Lori."*

But, it's true. I was painfully shy, and just as painfully insecure.

Moreover, because the kids I chose to share the majority of my time with didn't share my belief in God, it was quite a rare occasion if the subject was brought up at all.

I certainly made no plans to bring up the *God* conversation on my own.

Nonetheless, my Christianity was frequently brought to the attention of my friends simply due to the fact that whenever anyone would visit my home, evidence was not only *visible*, but *audible* as well, that ours was a Christian home.

One could not meet my parents or my siblings and not see and hear that our home was Christ-centered.

We had Bibles in just about every room in our home, along with other Bible-related reading and study materials. We had Scripture references on plaques on the walls. We went to church meetings every Sunday morning and every Sunday evening, and even on Wednesday nights for prayer meeting.

The youth group would often be invited over to our house after the Sunday evening church service for a *singspiration*, as we called it in those days. It was a time for the youth to sing praises to Jesus and have fellowship together with other teen believers.

We frequently had Bible readings and discussions as a family around our kitchen table after the dinner table was cleared in the evenings, with my father leading the study and discussion time. If you were a guest for dinner at our house, you were also included and encouraged to actively participate in the after-dinner Bible study.

My family and I participated in all this, among many other Christ-centered activities and events.

Thus, my friends' inquiring minds would often get the best of them which, in turn, required lots of answers from me - yes, me - perhaps their only real connection at that time to anything resembling religion.

Imagine that!

Me!

I was my friends' connectivity to Christianity.

Apparently, it's true what they say - the Lord really does work in mysterious ways.

STREET SMART KIDS

It's not so mysterious then, that I chose to befriend the *street smart kids*. Or, maybe it was the other way around. Perhaps it was them who chose to befriend me.

Whichever the case, we had a mutual understanding of each other that seemed to present itself with an extraordinary ease. I liked them, and they liked me. We were probably intrigued by one another.

And it may be that this mutual intrigue was part of God's master plan.

I'll bet it was! God really is a *know-it-all*. His plan is perfect. So is His timing.

I've been accused on much more than just one occasion of being quite naive.

But I prefer to think of myself not so much as naive as just pensively curious regarding the life events or intrinsic drives, or both, that *make people tick*, or that cause them to do the things they do.

Pursuance of my curiosity has caused me to discover that, contrary to popular belief, a surprisingly large number of *street smart kids* aren't necessarily as frightening as their appearances or actions may lead one to erroneously believe.

They may act tough on the outside, and may even dress the part. But it's nothing more than that - a dress rehearsal for the act of life.

Some are just better actors than others.

My own personal interactions with *street smart kids* over the years has taught me that they really do possess the same inborn needs as any other kids whether *rich* or *poor, shy* or *confident, Christian* or *atheist, smart* or *not-so-smart, athletic* or *musical,* or somewhere in between all those superlatives.

Street smart kids are just that ... smart on the street.

Why are they are *on the street* in the first place?

Who knows? There could be any number of reasons.

And, let's not even get into the game of placing blame on one thing or another, or one person or another. It really doesn't matter - at least not as far as having any relevance to the purpose of my story.

It is what it is.

And no matter the road that led them to their corner of the world/their place on the street - they are where they are.

That being said, it is a misconception of many teenagers that if they befriend the *street smart kids* - that will ensure their own safety on the street.

Just because a teenager is *street smart*, that does not in any way, shape or form translate into the teen being a safety net.

Street smarts are learned behaviors resulting from any number of possible teaching methods, or self-taught lessons.

When I speak of my own personal interactions with teenagers – *street smart* or otherwise - I am not simply referring those interactions that took place during my teenage years. I am referring also to those interactions that began long before I became a teenager, as well as to those that have continued fairly routinely ever since.

My sister and brother are ten and eight years older than me, respectively. So, from an early age, I have been surrounded by teenagers.

Additionally, for the greater part of my life I have made it my choice to continue to enjoy the company of teenagers. They can be a lot of fun!

Yes, they can!

As a small child there were always teenage friends of my sister and brother around the house.

I loved it.

When I became a teenager myself, I surrounded myself with my peers.

I loved it.

I became a mother while I was a teenager, so when my children became teenagers - especially my firstborn - I was still quite young.

I loved it.

Several years ago, I chose to start - not just take part in, but *start* - a program at the local high school educating teenagers about health occupations/careers. I *chose* to work with teenagers.

I loved it.

In my current career as a registered nurse, I have always preferred the opportunities to work with teenagers as compared with other age groups.

I love it.

Our youngest daughter frequently has teenage friends over to the house to visit.

I'm still loving it.

As for me, working with, talking with, and befriending teenagers is a little slice of Heaven right here on Earth. Well - most of the time.

No! I am not kidding.

A mountain of life lessons can be gathered from the teenager.

Likewise, if you give them the benefit of the doubt, very often they are more than willing to guzzle and absorb any and all *life's lessons* speeches spoken to them by an adult who genuinely cares for their well-being (even if they don't or won't admit it).

It is my choice and my pleasure to remain young-at-heart today, with no intention of ever changing the age or attitude of my heart.

Perhaps I am an unusual character as it regards forever holding a special place in my heart for teenagers. That's okay. I have never been described as *usual* anyways. And, I'm okay with that too.

All I am saying is, give teenagers a chance.

Given the chance, any kid really can be anything his or her heart desires.

Not given the chance ... well, that might be the time we need to begin seeking to place blame.

On the other hand, if a teenager willingly chooses not to take the chances or opportunities that are handed to him or her, he or she has no one to blame but him or herself.

Keep in mind though that if you give a teenager a chance and an opportunity, you might not see the positive results of your efforts until many years down the road.

Be patient.

Good things come to those who wait.

My own parents waited patiently for me.

Thanks, Mom and Dad.

Take a chance on a teenager. The final outcome just might surprise you, enlighten you, and give you a sense of satisfaction like nothing you could have dreamed.

Oh ... my skeleton?

That would be my pregnancy at sixteen young, teenage years of age.

Sixteen!

So young!

But, it all turned out okay *in the end* as they say.

Recall, if you will, our previous discussion about endings – the bright light at the end of the tunnel, and the rainbow at the end of the storm.

That being said, make permanent mental note that my skeleton is <u>not</u> my son, Danny.

Furthermore, use that same permanent marker to note that Danny's significance in my life is my own personal bright light and rainbow.

It's simply the pregnancy out of wedlock that haunts me, having forced me to close that heavy door that exposed my indiscretions.

It was not because I was embarrassed about the pregnancy (those days are gone), nor was it because I felt as though God didn't forgive me (He is always faithful to forgive when we ask for His forgiveness).

Rather, I kept my pregnant skeleton a secret because of those numerous adults who seem to *SCREAM* ruthless, persistent negativities about unwed, teenage mothers. Relentlessly! And, I just did not want to deal with any of that.

Of course, people knew that I had a son. It was just the history behind it all that I kept a secret.

C'mon! I was only sixteen years old. And, although I was beaming with pride about Danny, I struggled with self-esteem issues.

Like most teenagers who carry burdens associated with these struggles, I tried (successfully sometimes, I think) to hide my low self-esteem from anyone and everyone.

At long last however, I have made a determined decision to for here-ever-after deal confidently and directly with any and all persistently ruthless *screamers* of negativities against unwed teenage girls who are either pregnant or have been pregnant in the past.

It has been many, many years since I have been described as a quiet person. (Yes, there really was a time in my life when I was particularly bashful.)

And, although I have no intention of at any time participating in a scream-fest with the *screamers*, prepare your mind that throughout the remainder of this text I will be making my written *voice* heard loud, clear, and with a straightforwardness that has become the *new me*.

To shed a bit more light on the *old me*: I used to be secretive and quite ashamed of my former self – the unwed, pregnant teenager. No matter how many years had come and gone, I still would always consider my inner self to be nothing more than *that unwed, pregnant teenage girl*.

The *new me* – and it took thirty-five years to unlock the door to the new me, and then drag her out of hiding by the way – has resolved to speak loudly, boldly, frankly, and lovingly in defense of every solitary teenage soul out there … boy or girl, pregnant or not pregnant, low or no self esteem, or whatever teenage adversities lacerate their precious souls.

With all the sincerity I can muster, and from the bottom of my heart, I wish it had not taken so many tortuous years for me to finally open my mouth – wide.

But now that I have pried it open, my plan is to keep it open until I take my last breath, purposefully for this cause.

The *new me* has chosen to no longer be ashamed of any mistakes I have made, but rather to admit, *"Yes, I made some mistakes but, that's just what they were – mistakes – and, I have admitted my guilt, forgiven myself, accepted God's forgiveness, and am moving onward and upward in an effort to keep others from harboring guilt which only breeds shame and seemingly endless depression."*

Since I found myself pregnant at just sixteen years old in what seemed like the blink of an eye, I realized that I was going to have to grow up – much more rapidly than I had envisioned.

I mean, this was not at all my plan for my life.

It certainly was not what I dreamed of and hoped for when I was a little girl.

My hopes and dreams were not unlike the dreams of many little girls.

Besides every girl's fantasy of meeting prince charming and becoming his longed-for princess with whom I'd live happily-ever-after, I had somewhat more realistic dreams such as becoming perhaps a veterinarian, a lawyer, a missionary in an underdeveloped country, or even a nurse.

One of my dreams eventually did come true, but only after many years of soul searching followed by a powerful determination to prove to myself and others that I had the capability of becoming whomever and whatever I chose to become.

My dream that eventually developed into a reality was that of becoming a registered nurse.

In 1993, I graduated from nursing school.

This was after fifteen years of marriage (to Joe – to whom I have now been married for thirty-two years as of this writing), three children (the youngest of which was six months old when I entered nursing school), and years of harboring a self-esteem low enough to talk myself into the false belief that *"I'm just not smart enough to do anything other than be a good wife and mother"*.

Flashing back now to the sixteenth year of life, and to hopefully help you understand a little more clearly how instantaneously the unwed, teen pregnancy changed my life, imagine pushing the fast forward button on your DVD player, except that you're not simply fast forwarding a movie – rather, you are fast forwarding your life.

That's how it was for me.

To facilitate the formation of an even-clearer visualization of the enormity of my high-speed time travel into adulthood, I believe it's necessary for me to point out that my *DVD player* just entirely skipped over some parts of *my own personal movie* that I should have been able to experience, but regrettably did not.

You know - things like the prom, graduating with my friends (instead of with the kids a year ahead of me in school), the high school senior trip, senior skip day with my friends, a college experience, maybe veterinary school, maybe law school, maybe missionary training, possibly sharing an apartment with friends … those kinds of things, among others.

Oh, if we could only go back. Right?

Pay close attention now. Here's a little fast-forwarding of my life for you ...

Recognizing, at the age of sixteen years, that the course of my life was going to take a completely different direction than I had imagined, it became quite apparent that I was going to need to follow a new *map* of sorts.

So, I took summer high school courses during my pregnancy, which allowed me to graduate from high school a year early.

I received my high school diploma in June, 1975 when Danny was eight months old.

That autumn, I attended a business college for a year to get my secretarial degree.

After business college, I went to work full-time.

So, when the friends I grew up with were just graduating from high school, I was entering the work force.

Immediately upon graduation from business bollege in the spring of 1976, I landed a job as a legal secretary for a law firm in Toledo, Ohio.

Many thanks, by the way, to the five attorneys in that office for the opportunity to work there; but particularly to Dwight for having faith in me and for giving me the opportunity to prove to myself that I could work full-time while raising my child, as a single teenage parent.

I still had a lot to learn.

And, Dwight was a genuinely kindhearted gentleman, and gracious teacher of sorts.

Aside from my entry into the world of motherhood while still a child myself, this job proved to be for me a further nudge into the world of adulthood.

Remember, I was still only a teenager - just eighteen by this time.

In December of 1976, I met my husband, Joe.

Joe was not yet a Christian when I met him, but I introduced him to the Lord.

A few months after that introduction, he got saved during his college spring break trip to Daytona Beach, Florida.

This was not at all his original plan. Originally, his plan was to have a good ole time with good ole boys and girls at the beach.

I had a different plan for him. And I was hoping and praying that his trip to the beach would go according to *my* plan.

By this time in my life, and after all I had been through up to this point, I had made the decision to turn my life back over to Jesus, and to present the gospel of Christ to others with a renewed boldness.

Before Joe left for his trip, I added to his luggage a Bible and some gospel tracts, hoping that he would read them in his spare time.

I encouraged him to do so.

He did.

And, he asked the Lord into his heart during a Wednesday night prayer meeting at a Baptist church in Daytona Beach.

I was more than thrilled.

I was falling in love, and now this man was a fellow believer in Jesus Christ.

Joe and I were engaged the following spring, and married in January, 1978.

When we had been married for just six months, we moved from a small apartment in my hometown to an even smaller apartment in Joe's hometown.

I thought this was going to be great, essentially because people didn't know me there. And, I was more than just okay with that.

Why?

Why not?

Being an *unknown* meant that I would not have to bear the burden of being constantly reminded of my own *history*, unless I chose to open those *history* books myself to share only with those folks who might be understanding and accept me for not only who I had become, but for who I had been.

It was such a good feeling for me to be able to *lock up my skeleton*, and maybe even throw away the key.

Indeed, I felt that by disposing of that wicked key, I would finally be given the chance to break free from the mold that other folks who *"knew me when"* just kept trying with all their might to push me into, with no means of escape.

But this, I thought, would be the perfect *escape*.

Little did I know, and didn't figure out for myself until many years down the road that *locking up my skeleton* was *bad for business* – the *business* of taking the best emotional care of myself.

We bought our first home in Joe's hometown.

It was a big old house – around one hundred years old - on Main Street.

It used to belong to the town physician back when the streets were nothing more than dirt.

It needed some work, but we loved it.

To me, it was picturesque. Storybook, almost.

Our new home place had a big old-fashioned front porch where we could sit on cool spring, warm summer, and chilly autumn evenings while visiting with the neighbors or watching the kids ride their bicycles down the sidewalks which were lined with beautiful shade trees that seemed to have been there forever.

There was a country church around the corner, and another country church just down the road.

The doctor's office was within walking distance, as well as the grocery store, the dime store, and the pizza shop.

Danny could walk or ride his bicycle to school, ride his bicycle to baseball practices and games, and walk to the corner store to get a *"mystery"* ice cream cone with his buddies, David and Clay, for a nickel. Yep – just a nickel.

The *"mystery"* ice cream cone was simply a cone filled with whatever flavor of ice cream or mixture of ice creams that were left at the bottom of the container(s). The kids loved it. I think they thought it was particularly special just because it had the word *mystery* in it.

I loved it because it was a cheap treat for the kids.

And, we surely didn't have much money to our names back then.

On lazy summer afternoons, Danny would often come into the house to grab his fishing pole and tackle box in order to go fishing in the creek that ran just behind our house.

We had a half-acre lot, and the creek was at the back of the lot.

Perfect!

I can still picture Danny sitting on the rickety old wooden bridge that crossed the creek, patiently waiting for a fish to take the bait.

It didn't seem to matter to Danny whether he fished alone or with friends. He just really liked to fish. Still does!

Frequently, in the late afternoons after Joe would get home from work, he and Danny would once again throw their fishing poles over their shoulders, tackle boxes in hand, and walk to the nearby pond to fish some more.

By this time, Joe had adopted Danny as his own son. And hey, that's what dads and sons do, they fish together, which has the very real potential of leading to great father/son bonding.

I gave birth to our second child while living in this quaint little town, a little sister for Danny.

Shannon Leanne was born when Danny was eight years old.

He adapted to the job of big brother with an ease that was nothing short of amazing.

He's still an awesome brother, to two sisters now.

His littlest sister, Shelby, was born when he was fifteen years old.

We lived in our charming little town until 1985, when Danny and Shannon were ten and two years old, respectively.

More than likely, we would still be living in the same town and in the same home if it hadn't been for the opportunity given to Joe to make a better living elsewhere.

So, we packed up the kids and whatever meager belongings we had and moved.

Our next home was in North Carolina.

People didn't know any of us at all there.

And, if people assumed that Joe was Danny's biological father, that was just fine and dandy with me.

I was quite comfortable with the idea of allowing people to assume whatever they chose.

As a matter of fact, I became lovingly accustomed to the normality of having folks make their fairy tale assumptions about our little family.

And if anyone ever said to me, *"Wow you started having children early,"* my well-rehearsed reply was simply, *"Yes, I did."* Or better yet, *"Yes, we did."*

Conversation over.

From time to time, however, I'd run full-face into women (*only* women, because men characteristically just don't think too deeply about, or waste their energies on, the *gossip-driven* stories that women seem to take great pleasure in) who just could not and would not let the sleeping dog remain in dream land.

Their ruthless determination to wake up that very tired dog (me), or to search relentlessly for my teenage skeleton key, was more than I could emotionally bear.

If I had to choose only one thing that irritates the living daylights out of me, it is the busybody who has to know everything - every detail – and then, spreads the gossip to her buddies.

She'll tell you she doesn't *repeat* gossip. So, you better be certain to listen carefully the first time.

Somebody once told me that she never lets the truth get in the way of a good story.

Be on your guard. She and those of like mind could be lurking in your own backyard digging up the *dirt* on you.

I was pregnant with Danny back in the day when abortion had just recently been legalized. Therefore, many young girls in a situation like mine either got an abortion, or they gave their babies up for adoption.

Never having been accused of being a follower, neither of those two options appealed to me.

I wanted my baby.

Really!

So, I chose to take a leadership role, making my own choice to carry my baby to full term and be his mother.

I proudly named him Danny Lee.

Yep! I took responsibility for my situation and made my own path.

You might be thinking, *"Leader, my foot!"* And possibly even, *"She was a master at playing follow the leader with the kids she chose to befriend."*

Ah, to the contrary!

Allow me to clarify, setting the record straight.

I liked to spread myself around, and hang with a vast variety of teenagers.

As a matter of fact, it didn't matter to me which group I was with, I made friends with all of them. No matter which group of kids I chose to hang with at a given moment, I was not one of the many followers. Rather, I preferred to take a leadership role, and if not a leader, then an able assistant to their cause.

I'll take this even a step or more further.

I genuinely liked everybody, and wanted to be everybody's friend. And, I wanted them to like me too, and to consider me a good friend.

Like all teenagers, I wanted to *fit in*.

And in my particular case, I wanted something even more. I wanted to fit in *everywhere* with *everyone*.

So, I made it my business to modify my character according to which group of friends I was choosing to hang out with at any given time.

For instance:

- Within the *smart* crowd, I was the *not so smart* kid.
- Within the *not so smart* crowd, I was the *smart* kid.
- Within the *athletic* crowd, I was the fan.
- Within the *musical* crowd, I was the encourager.
- Within the *introverted* crowd, I was the noisy one/the prankster.
- Within the *extroverted* crowd, I was the prankee.
- Within the *street smart* crowd, I was the one to be protected.
- Within the *Christian* crowd, I was the lost soul.

Despite my having given in to my sinful nature (we're all born with it, by the way), God blessed me with Danny.

The blessing of Danny's birth was the beginning of a positive change for the betterment of me.

God is still hard at work in molding and shaping me to conform to His perfect plan for my life. I am ever-changing, ever-learning, and keenly aware that God is not finished with me yet.

One of my favorite quotes that I frequently heard from my father is, *"It takes a lifetime of living to learn how to live."* Now, ain't that the truth!

No, I wasn't a *bad* girl. Like so many other teenagers before me and after me, I was just a confused teenage girl, looking for love and acceptance … and, learning how to live.

To those parents who wanted to keep their daughters and sons away from me because I might be a *bad influence,* and who looked at me like I should be ashamed … perhaps your shameful fingers are pointed in the wrong direction.

Just because my own poor judgment was out in the open (you can't hide a pregnant belly for very long), it did not make me any more of a sinner than those who *cover up* their poor judgment by having an abortion.

Oddly, it's a rare occasion to hear negativities being whispered about the gal who sucked away the life of her child.

Even more rarely are voices heard criticizing the very hands that operate the suction equipment.

Have you ever wondered why it is that no one talks negatively about *those* girls and those *so-called* medical providers?

The answer to that question is no secret – it's obvious, in fact. It's because their sins are *hidden*. They are *hidden* just like the sins of the *boy* who participates in sex outside of marriage, and like the sins of the *adult* who partakes in an extramarital affair.

Just because we can't *see* those sins in the same manner that we can *see* the sins of the pregnant teenage girl, that doesn't make them any less of a sin.

"You who are without sin cast the first stone." (Read the story about the adulteress in *John 8: 1-11.)*

Let me make one more thing crystal clear. I am by no means throwing stones at the young ladies and women that have had abortions in the past, nor at those who will sadly choose to have abortions in the future.

Though I have never traveled down the abortion road myself, God knows I have my own sins with which to concern myself.

To those who have aborted their babies, my prayer is that you will, or that you already have, come to the realization that this - like my out-of-wedlock experience - is a sin against God.

Though the abortion may be hidden for a while, at some time its memory will make its ugly reappearance and must be dealt with by repentance.

After repentance and the forgiveness of God, one must also forgive herself.

And, it is my understanding from post-abortion survivors, that forgiveness of self is a very long, very lonesome, and very tortuous road to recovery.

But, you *can* do it!

If you have had an abortion, my heart goes out to you in the most genuine way. Though what you have done is wrong *according to God's Holy Word* - God is faithful and just to forgive you. You only need to genuinely repent, and simply ask.

Your sin is no worse than any other.

Always remember that. Just as a rose by any other name is still a rose, a sin by any other name is still just that - a sin.

According to God's Holy Word, sin does not have categories or sub-sets or ratings. It's either sinful or sinless. It's either black or white. There is no gray area.

The abortionist is not without sin either. Let alone the fact that he/she apparently pays no mind to his/her sacred oath taken upon entry into the world of *doctorhood* to *"do no harm."*

The harm they cause to the little lives they abruptly end is nothing less than brutal, nothing less than horrendous, and nothing less than pure evil.

Have you taken the time to intently investigate the horror endured by the victim - the baby - during the abortion procedure?

Man up! Look it up.

But, be aware that the task set before you - digging up photos and videos and in-depth reading material - will be far from easy to find. Anything *but* easy.

Why?

Through my own such investigations, I have learned that this is apparently due to the fact that most resources (e.g., the internet) claim that the material is too *"graphic"*.

They're right. It *is* graphic.

But, it is also reality.

It's not just that the beating heart is stopped (as awful as that is), or that some miscellaneous tissue is removed, as some would make you believe.

The sickening, gut-wrenching reality is that in most cases, the life is ripped limb by precious limb. And the photographs of the end result are nothing less than horrifying. It's worse than any horror movie I've ever seen.

What kind of sick mind participates in inflicting this upon anyone at all, but an innocent child?

Child molesters have nothing on the abortionist.

Get your vomit bag ready.

I personally know of many women who have had abortions. They come from both sides of the abortion debate.

Some are very young, and some much older. Some are girls from my high school days, and some are former high school students of my own. Some are churched, some are unchurched. Some regret what they have done, some will come to regret it much further down the road of life.

But, not one of them had the abortion because of health reasons.

No. These ladies had their abortions either for the sake of *convenience*, or because they were terribly *frightened*.

In case you feel somewhat confused about what might be so frightening for an unwed, pregnant young lady that it causes her to seek an abortion – you might want to review my discussion earlier about *SCREAMERS*, as well as other plights of teen motherhood previously discussed.

Many of these friends and acquaintances who played a painful part in the termination of their babies' lives, were so young that I believe them when they tell me they didn't really know what they were doing at the time, but that they were just *"scared."*

In these cases, the abortionist apparently didn't deem it necessary to fully explain the procedure - let alone its agonizing mental disturbances *further down the road of life* to these ladies - even though he or she took that sacred *oath*.

These young girls were not *MIS*informed.

They were *UN*informed.

On the flip side, others knew exactly what they were doing at the time and did it anyway.

Statistics have shown that less than one percent of abortions are for health reasons. That thought bears repeating for the sake of emphasis.

Less than one percent!

I've always been a great deal more than merely curious about this statistic. It just was not specific enough for me.

Health reasons? I wondered, *"What health reason would warrant an abortion?"*

So, I asked some doctors at random. Not doctors with whom I worked, but doctors with whom I had become otherwise acquainted.

Some folks have said to me, *"Geez, Lori - don't you think that's a little bold to ask such a question of those who perform the abortions?"*

Bold?

Nope. Just clued-in and on-my-toes!

I've always considered the *horse's mouth* my best resource.

Not surprisingly, the responses that I was given by those doctors who took *"the oath"* without intent to respect it were mind-grippingly unanimous.

Their comebacks were undivided that if the mother was distraught by the pregnancy, then an abortion would be the *healthy* procedure required for the mental sake of the mother.

I am well aware that there have been cases where the mother's life might truly be at great risk if a pregnancy is carried forward.

These are rare instances. Look it up. See for yourself.

And I am certain these are instances wherein the parents are tormented and distraught about the situation. My heart genuinely goes out to them.

That being said, I can only speak for myself when I declare with 100 percent assuredness that if I were in any such situation, I would give up my life in order to spare the life of my child. My family and good friends have heard me make this remark repeatedly for the past thirty-five years. I have not wavered.

If you have had an abortion in the past, I am praying for you daily.

Really, I am!

If you are considering an abortion now, my plea is that you will not do it.

Instead, at least carry your baby to full term.

It will not ruin your life. But, abortion will bring to ruin the chance for life of one who cannot speak for himself/herself.

Anything that gives life is worth any conceived notion of temporary inconvenience. In the grand scheme of things, any such inconvenience is so short term. And, there are so many options other than abortion.

Pregnancy is only nine short months of your life.

I chose life for my son, Danny.

Not once have I regretted that decision.

Not once!

Thank God I don't have to deal with the torment of having had an abortion.

My prayer for those of you who have is that you will ask God for forgiveness, and then know that his forgiveness is permanent, and He will give you the peace that passes all understanding.

If you are considering abortion, or if you have had an abortion, please allow me to encourage you to see wise Christian counseling. There are many communities across the United States and Canada that have a pregnancy care center to help you with your tough situation and to provide you with direction and alternatives.

So, if you don't feel like you can go to a parent or a friend or even your preacher with your own *secret*, please know that you can go to a pregnancy care center and receive confidential help and information.

When I was a little girl in Sunday school, we used to sing a song about Heaven that included the words, *"The seats are filling fast in my Father's house."*

I loved that song. I believe however, that Heaven's seats have been filling entirely too fast over the past thirty-six or more years, since abortion has become a *legal crime*.

Too many precious little lives are literally being *sucked out* of existence, unable to make their voices heard or their wishes known.

Though these precious, innocent children have been and continue to be gruesomely destroyed and disposed of before being allowed to experience the joys of childhood here on Earth, God has never and will never allow their disposal to destroy their opportunity to experience everlasting enjoyment with Him.

Their eternal home now is in Heaven – safe in the arms of Jesus.

No one can *rip apart* that relationship.

To those of you who remain compelled to do some stone throwing, consider this: The teenager that you're so vindictive about today just might be your next-door neighbor in Heaven tomorrow. In fact, even I might be your next-door neighbor in Glory someday.

We've all experienced the world of adolescence.

Let us be ever mindful of our own past poor judgments, mistakes, and challenges.

We've all been in that place. If you're still young and in the adolescent world at this moment, know that there'll be ups and downs your entire life, but you have the opportunity right now and every day to create for yourself more ups than downs.

PART TWO

CHALLENGES

CHAPTER THREE
ADOLESCENCE

*"The fear of The Lord is the beginning of knowledge,
But fools despise wisdom and instruction."*
Proverbs 1: 7

Teenagers don't live on Easy Street.

Most commonly, their place of residence is on Confusion Boulevard with *opposing lanes of traffic* on either side of the greener grass lining the middle of the road.

And though the greener grass would appear to be just footsteps away, it seems to require walking miles upon miles in teenage shoes in order to reach the lush contentment that the greenery affords.

Confusion reigns within the soul that houses the teenager.

Though some teens might turn on the false air of confidence that seems to radiate dignity and grace while dealing with raging hormones and body changes (desired or undesired), confusion is king in their land.

The teenager's homeland – his or her soul – is quite often overrun with what may appear to some as pandemonium.

At least, it contains all the ingredients necessary in a recipe for emotional upset.

Some teenagers throw all these ingredients into the mix haphazardly, unmethodically, and without measurement; while other teenagers seem more apt to measure precisely (or thereabout), being a little more certain of the resulting table set before them.

Not me!

I was more prone to being pandemonized by my own soul.

Measure the ingredients of my daily ins, outs, and whereabouts? Are you kidding? I didn't have time for that.

I just threw all my ingredients, which often consisted of chaos and mayhem, into the pot and turned my internal stove on the highest setting.

After all, I was a teenager.

I had things to do, places to go, people to see. My life was waiting for me. And not very patiently, I might add. Or at least, I did not want to wait for *it*.

Measure?

Nope. Time was a-wastin'.

It's sad now looking back at a large portion of my teenage years. Time wasn't wasting away at all. But, I was pretty good at wasting time.

I didn't realize then what I realize now - that time was my friend. Time was on my side.

Time should have been the main ingredient in the casserole that I call my life.

But, I just couldn't resist the *express* way of life. You know, for the same reason that we have drive-through fast food restaurants. We want our piece of the pie, and we want it now.

I think I might have wanted the whole pie, or at least a taste of the assortment.

If law enforcement officials were authorized to give teenagers tickets for driving in the fast lane of life, I probably would have had enough citations to cause them to revoke my life license.

But, there is no such law.

So, I just kept driving on that twisted highway which would ultimately lead to my teenage pregnancy and teen motherhood.

In fact, the more I think about it, the more I think maybe my quick trip through adolescence was more like a non-stop flight to adulthood.

It was not round trip.

My ticket took me directly to adulthood and left me there.

Confusion vs. Confidence. That's the wrestling match teenagers routinely attend – whether they want to or not.

Confidence enters the ring tapping the teen on one shoulder exerting all rationalizing effort to convince the teen, *"You can do it".*

Confusion, on the other hand (or shoulder) enters on the irrational side of the ring not tapping but pounding the opposite shoulder while screaming, *"No, you can't".*

Confusion just won't let up. Its attempts to beat the teenager down are relentless. *Confusion* is mean. *Confusion* is cocky. And, *Confusion* is sneaky.

It's like that wolf in sheep's clothing. It makes relentless attempts to persuade the teenager to make some awfully big mistakes in the ring of life that have the potential of leaving lifetime scars.

Not all teenagers throw in the towel. But, many teens do just stop and give that towel a defeated toss.

Confusion is a fierce competitor.

Those of us who have survived the sometimes tortuous teenage years, and maybe have even come out on top, have the awesome opportunity to take delight in helping the teenagers of today realize their potential and individuality.

I am by no means saying that counseling the teenager is always delightful. Far from it sometimes. But it is well worth the effort - in the end, as they say.

Potentially, the delightfulness of it all may not be seen for days, or weeks, or even years.

Someday isn't always *just around the corner.* Just ask my mom and dad.

My *corner* took a quite some time to reach. Indeed, it was an awfully long walk.

I am confident that I am not just speaking for myself when I remark, *"The world was confusing to me as a teenager."*

We've all *been there.*

Yes, you were!

On top of that, I'm not so certain that we ever become totally un-confused.

Rather, it is my strong belief that we sometimes allow ourselves to become complacent, and even detached or unaware - unaware of potential defects or dangers in our society.

I might be taking a stab in the dark here, but I have a sneaking suspicion that the generation before mine (e.g., my mom and dad's generation - he was born in 1927 and she in 1928) were more on the ball regarding the government, politics, and current issues when compared with young adults today.

See for yourself if I'm right here or not. Ask several individuals who are currently in their twenties, questions about our Country, politics, government, and current issues in the news. Tough questions.

I presuppose that many, if not most, will not be able to answer tough questions.

Complacency?

You betcha.

Who taught them that?

Think about it.

The generation before mine also seemed to be a lot more on the ball regarding raising children to be responsible adults.

I know. There are exceptions to every rule. But generally speaking, my parents' generation didn't seem to have had such a tough time with teaching and reinforcing to their kids rules, guidelines, and expectations.

Their generation was determined too, that children would be well-prepared for life outside the comforts of home when they reached adulthood.

Presently, many kids who are entering college don't even have the first clue what they want to do with their life. They're still *"thinking about it."*

Didn't they already have eighteen years to *think* about it? Maybe that's why we still call them *kids* when they enter college. When I was their age ...

Never mind!

Do you want to really learn some things? The really *important* things? The things that really *matter* in life?

No, you don't have to take a college class. Simply take the time to talk, and especially listen, to someone from my mom and dad's era. No - make the time. Before it's too late.

We should've listened when we were teenagers. And, we should be wise enough to pass that knowledge along to our own teenagers.

You might be thinking, *"Okay then, if Lori's mom and mad were so in tune with parenting and knew so much, why was Lori so confused?"*

For the same reason all teenagers are confused.

Life.

Let's consider just *some* of the things that make life so confusing to the teenager ...

- You're expected to automatically act like an adult - when it seems like you were just a child yesterday.
- You WERE just a child yesterday!
- You wake up one morning, and presto! Everyone is telling you to act your age.
- You ARE acting your age!
- You have to wash up, clean up, and dress up - but, can't act up.
- You think you're in love.
- You think you're in love again - and, again - and, again.
- You get dumped by your boyfriend/girlfriend.
- You have to figure out how to dump your boyfriend/girlfriend.
- You GET to learn how to drive.
- You HAVE to get a job so that you can get gas so that you can drive.
- You have to get good grades so that you can get into a good college.
- Who's got time for studying to get the good grades when there are so many social activities to keep up with?
- You want the best of things when you grow up.
- You don't want to grow up; and you want those best things NOW.
- Sex? Weren't you just playing with trucks or dolls yesterday - on the playground?
- Life is coming at you fast. Too fast!

And ...

- Why do some people have functional families, while others have dysfunctional families?

- Why do some people die young, while others die at a *ripe old age?*
- Why do some people stay married, while others *can't get it right the first time?*
- Why do some people have talents, while others have none?
- Why do some families have money, while other families have so little or no income?
- Why do some families go to church, while others stay home and watch television?
- Why are there good neighborhoods and bad neighborhoods? –

Doesn't everyone want to live in a good neighborhood?

- Why are there so many different religions, and so many different churches to choose from?
- Why are some people fat, while others are starving?

- Why do some people discipline their kids, while other kids "get away with everything?"
- Why do some parents make a big deal about lying and cheating, yet they make this part of *their* daily routine?

Let alone the infamous ...

- *"Who am I, and why am I here"?*

WHY are teenagers so confused? *WHY NOT?*

No, teenagers don't live on Easy Street.

Rather, the winding paths they travel to get to Destination Road can be quite rough and bumpy.

CHAPTER FOUR
PEER PRESSURE

*"Do you not know that friendship with the world
Is enmity with God? Whoever therefore wants to be
A friend of the world makes himself an enemy of God."
James 4: 4*

Why do all teenagers look alike and act alike?
They don't. Remember? We've been over this already in detail, back in Chapter 2.

Sure, they may be somewhat similar on the outside, causing them to be easily identifiable as a teenager.

Maybe they even wear their hair in similar fashion, or prefer clothing that is acceptable within their own peer groups.

They have no wrinkles and no gray hair.

And, invariably, they even have their own language and typical gestures.

But within each group there are different characters. And each character has developed his or her own individuality of sorts.

We've talked a little bit about this already, too.

Think about the television shows your teenager watches for instance -the ones with teenagers *in* them.

The kids in those shows aren't all alike. They each have very distinctive traits, styles, and personalities reflecting their own individuality.

- happy
- sad
- tall
- short
- fat
- skinny
- comedian
- sob-story teller
- good-looking
- not-so-good looking
- coordinated
- uncoordinated
- respectful
- disrespectful
- compliant
- non-compliant
- organized
- disorganized
- decisive
- indecisive
- leader
- follower
- talented

- untalented
- friendly
- not-so-friendly
- talkative
- quiet
- dare devil
- timid
- in shape
- out of shape
- healthy
- unhealthy
- rich
- poor
- functional home life
- dysfunctional home life
- only child
- one of several children

Get the idea?

That list could go on *from here 'til kingdom come*, as my mom used to say. But, I think you've got the picture.

Could it be that sometimes we just don't take the time to look beyond that first glance, beyond that first impression, and beyond the *outer layer* that envelopes the teenager?

Apparently.

That *outer layer* doesn't define a teenager anymore than the *blanket of adulthood* defines who you really are.

Kids don't want to be just a reproduction of one another. They just want to be *with* one another, just like you and I prefer to identify with those folks in our own age group.

And, even though you and I might share some similarities with those our own age, that doesn't mean that everyone in our own age group is just like us.

I have no doubt that there are some of you my own age reading this book even now and thinking, *"Lori is nothing like me."* Additionally, I would venture to say that some of you may prefer not even to join me for dinner if asked - simply because of our *inner* differences.

We, like the teenagers, tend to find our place in this world with those who are likeminded.

Teenagers are likeminded in this way - they all just want to fit in ... somewhere. Thus, the unmediated and unavoidable formation of peer groups - even for you.

What makes someone a peer anyways?

- someone who shares your interests
- someone who holds the same beliefs as you
- someone you admire
- someone you respect
- someone your age

Throughout the entirety of our lives, we choose to associate with our peers.

Then, why do we feel this so-called peer *pressure*?

Where in the world did that come from?

Perhaps its birth was due to our own impression that maybe those in our peer group, or other peer groups for that matter, *had it all*. I personally believe that to be the case in the majority of instances.

And what specifically is *"all"*?

For the teenager, *all* might be a lot or it might not be much. *All* could be love, or popularity, or excitement, or money, or good grades, or friends, or happiness ... or, *all of the above.*

My dad always used to say, *"Lori, don't believe anything you hear, and only half of what you see."*

It took awhile for me to recognize the significance of that quote. But, now that I have identified its implication, I wish there were some way to implant a little transmitter into the minds of the teenagers whereby we as parents could empower them with the understanding that everything is not always what it appears to be.

Case in point - From time to time I've had folks (who *think* they know me) remark *"Lori, you're so lucky."*

Lucky?

Down on my luck sometimes, maybe. But, not lucky.

Oh, no! Not by any stretch of the imagination. These people do not know me as well as they think they do.

Falling down, and picking yourself up by your bootstraps is not lucky.

Its perseverance.

Being stomped on by somebody else's boots, and getting back into the ring of life is not lucky.

Its strength to go on.

I've fallen a lot. Over and over again, in fact.

And, I've been the *stomping ground* for others a lot. So much so that my *stomping ground stories* could be another entire book.

If we were to sit down together, I could tell you story upon story of my *unluckiness*. There are so many stories that you would likely be dumbfounded by the enormity of it all. But, I press on. God gives me the strength to do so.

And, if you've walked in shoes that look like mine – and I speculate that the majority of folks reading this story have probably worn similar shoes - God is able to bestow that same strength upon you. All you have to do is ask, and walk side by side with Him. He can make your worn shoes new again.

And rest assured, when your shoes begin to have that shabby look again from time to time – and they will - give them to God. He'll make all the necessary repairs.

On the flip side of my unluckiness, I will whole heartedly say that I am blessed.

Undeservedly!

But, blessed just the same. Blessed beyond my dreams!

I have a fond remembrance of a high school teacher who once told me, *"Lori ... Stay close to God, and He will bless you beyond your dreams."*

He revealed this truth to me during my teen pregnancy. And, I've never forgotten it. In fact, it has replayed over and over again in my mind – *like a broken record*, as they say.

Why?

Because it works! And, because my dreams cannot compare with the blessings I have received from Jesus. And, all it takes is staying close to Him.

When I was pregnant with Danny, my Dad showed me a Scripture that has not only helped me tremendously; but, whenever I read it I am reminded of my Dad's love for me.

As a matter of fact, it made such an impression on me that I remember where I was sitting at the table in our kitchen when he read it to me for the first time.

Well ... he probably read it to me many times before, but evidently I wasn't listening.

He probably thought I wasn't listening this time either. But, I was.

You know, teenagers often appear to be not listening – but, they are.

I was.

I heard.

And, I remembered.

> *"One thing I do, forgetting those things which are behind and reaching forward to those things which are ahead, I press toward the goal for the prize of the upward call of God in Christ Jesus." – Philippians 3: 13-14*

What my dad was trying to get across to me by introducing me (or, re-introducing, as the case may be) to this Scripture is this: We all make mistakes. We all make errors in judgment. But, we cannot and should not let those things bring us down and keep us down forever. We must learn from our mistakes and pick ourselves right back up, and move on, move forward, never look back, forgive ourselves for any wrong doings, and forget about it. Just forget about beating ourselves up over these things.

Every one of us falls or fails at one time or another, but we can turn the tables on our failures and take the lessons we have learned from them to help others who may be struggling or falling in the same manner.

That's where the *"reaching forward to those things which are ahead"* and the *"pressing toward the goal for the prize of the upward call of God in Christ Jesus"* comes in.

In other words, we can use our failures for good by sharing not only the *failure* part of our story, but also by sharing how through it all God brought us to the other side – the *successful* side - by turning our lives over to Him and taking hold of His hand for divine guidance; and in turn, reaching out to others in order to let them know that they too can receive God's forgiveness and healing touch.

No, I will not go into detail in this book about the many times I've fallen, or even the manner in which I've been underneath someone else's boot, enduring strangulation – it's irrelevant - and, you can't move on if you don't let go.

What *is* relevant is that there is relevance to my life now. I continue to take daily, steady steps towards God's calling in my life to be there for anyone who now *is* where I once *was*.

Do I still fall sometimes?

Yep.

Do I still feel like I'm suffocating underneath the boot of someone else from time to time?

Yep.

Am I okay with that?

Not really! But, I deal with it - much better than I used to - and I move forward.

Regrettably, from time to time over the years I have found myself with my hand on the rewind button of my life, causing me to walk backward instead of forward, and beating myself up over it all - all over again.

I'm not necessarily off the track at those times, I'm just heading in the wrong direction.

And, at some point during my wayward travels, God allows something to happen in my life causing me to shift gears and move forward once again.

Life lessons are hard sometimes, but that's okay. I know how to pull myself up and dust myself off now.

And, that's the message I hope to convey through the pages of this book - this chapter of my life - that if I can do it, anybody can do it. Really, because there are an awful lot of *chapters* in my life, but those are other stories for another time.

One of my toughest life lessons was the pressure from peers and from within myself to have a boyfriend.

I didn't really know anything about true love.

Let me rephrase. During my adolescence I was certain I knew everything there was to know about true love, but now that those days are behind me I have come to realize that my love knowledge level was ... was ... *what love knowledge level?* I had none.

Nonetheless, peer pressure as well as my self-induced pressure to desire love (or what I mistakenly *thought* was love) from a young man - another teenager who didn't really know anything about love but just *thought* he did - ultimately placed me in a scary situation, a situation that shifted me from adolescence to adulthood in the blink of an eye.

Just a blink.

While getting ready for bed one night just like any average teenager, I looked at myself in the mirror and wondered what the next day would bring.

When I awoke the next morning, I still wondered.

But by that afternoon, I was no longer simply wondering what the next day would bring. No. By that afternoon it hit me. Hard!

In fact, I was now wondering what the next eighteen or so years would bring.

You see, that afternoon I was given the news that in just a few short teenage months I was going to be one of *"them."*

I was going to be somebody's *Mommy*.

CHAPTER FIVE
TEEN PREGNANCY

*"And be kind one to another, tenderhearted,
Forgiving one another,
Even as God in Christ forgave you."
Ephesians 4:32*

Though my memory may be *"dim"* on a number of things, I have a hundred-watt recollection of the moment that I found out that in just a few months someone, a very little someone, was going to be depending on me – *ME!* - for everything.

I was still dependent on my own parents. How was this going to work?

I remember this one moment in time as if it occurred only yesterday ...

My mom had just picked me up from high school. As she drove what turned out to be the longest drive home ever from school, I noticed that she was suspiciously quiet. I could tell that she was deep in thought, but I had the distinct feeling that she might share those deep thoughts with me.

She kept looking at me with those distinctively special *"mom eyes"*. You know - the mother's eyes that are so intensely loving, yet so intensely concerned at the same time.

I sensed that she must have something terribly important to tell me. It quickly became obvious to me that, at any moment, whatever was on her mind would be verbally passed along to me. She had something to say, something to tell me, but she just wasn't quite sure where to begin. I thought, *"Did somebody die?"*

As we were driving down the road, having already turned onto the quaint, midwestern street where we lived, my mom (who had taken me some days or weeks earlier to the family doctor for a pregnancy test – because moms really do seem to have a kind of sixth sense, especially about their own offspring) decided to just come out and say what I'm sure had been weighing quite heavily on her mind all day so far.

Ever so gently, compassionately, and quietly, but matter-of-factly, she put her precious hand in mine and said, *"Lori, you are pregnant."*

It was at that moment that my hundred-watts of mind juices really started flowing and in fact, went into overload.

My heart sank to my stomach.

Then, my stomach made its way up to my throat.

My once rosy cheeks now lacked of any color at all. My insuppressible tears flooded my cheeks, drenched my clothes, and sprinkled onto my high school books.

I glanced over at my mom again.

Her *"mom eyes"* were bigger-than-life filled with the compassion that only a mom can have for her child. In my case, a *child having a child* – her *baby having a baby*.

After swallowing the big lump in my throat (it took several attempts), I quietly asked my mom to *"just drive around the block"*.

I wasn't ready to go into the house yet.

I wasn't ready to go on with the rest of the afternoon.

Quite frankly, I wasn't ready for anything.

And, I sure wasn't ready to be a mommy. Not me. Not at sixteen!

Life for me, for a few moments, stood strangely still.

Somehow, I had to get a hold of myself and absorb this overwhelming piece of information that my mom had just shared with me. But no matter how hard I tried, it would not - could not - sink in. Or, perhaps it just sunk to the pits of my stomach.

My mom obliged my request to keep driving.

We took a slow, leisurely drive - but I'm quite certain my mom's thoughts were racing. I'm not sure if we just rode around the block, or if we went for a much longer drive.

I just sat there. Staring ... at nothing.

My mom was likely expressing her feelings of love for me, and telling me that somehow we would get through this, and that things would all work out. But, the more I thought - the more it seemed that someone was slowly lowering the dimmer switch connected to my mind juices.

Then - lights off.

I could no longer think.

I could barely breathe.

My mind simply could not absorb the complexity of it all.

Shock!

To this day, no matter how hard I might try. I cannot recall the remainder of that day - except for this ... this thing that still sends chills - good, heartwarming chills - all over my body.

My dad sat down with me. He started the conversation. Thank goodness! Because I could not have started a conversation no matter how hard I might have tried. I just did not know what to say. I wouldn't have known where to begin. If I had tried to open my mouth, I'm quite certain absolutely nothing would have come out. C'mon. I was just a kid. A kid having a kid.

My father, on the other hand, knew exactly what to say. And he said it so well ... so perfect ... so like a father who truly loves his daughter deeply and *unconditionally*.

His voice was soft, gentle, and heartfelt. The comforting words of my dear, devoted Daddy went something like this: *"Lori, I know what you've done. Your mom and I forgive you. And, we love you."*

Then, for what seemed like an eternity, he hugged me ... tight.

Together, we cried.

I have more love for my mom and my dad than my heart can hold.

Are you surprised at my mom and dad's response? You shouldn't be. I already told you how phenomenal they are.

The next tough step, among many more to come, was to tell Danny's biological father about my unexpected pregnancy. I did. He didn't seem particularly concerned. The solution, in fact, seemed pretty clear to him - abortion.

Sure – the *quick fix* or *the remedy* to the situation at hand.

Danny's biological father was my age. Just a young teenager himself. So, I'm certain the whole idea of causing a pregnancy was scary to him as well.

Abortion was legal now. It had been legal for about a year. And, *everyone was doing it.*

This young man's view of the situation was as opposite of mine as one can get.

He made it crystal clear that he had no intention of involving himself in caring about the situation at all.

He also made it clear that it was not at all *his* problem, but *mine.*

And to him, abruptly putting an end to the pregnancy - eliminating a life from existence - was the best choice, perhaps even the *only* choice.

I, on the other hand, could not justify ending a baby's life just because the circumstances surrounding this pregnancy were not ideal. In fact, under no circumstances was I going to have an abortion.

Abort the precious, innocent little life growing inside me?

Are you kidding me? Not a chance!

So - alone, I went forward with the pregnancy. Alone!

As I recall, Danny's biological father only called me on the telephone one time during the lonely months of my pregnancy. And, by his own choice, in-person visits never occurred.

Once in a while, we would see each other in passing, out in public - like at the mall or walking down the sidewalks in town. And, it was just that – *in passing*. I would barely get a nod hello from him, if that - no words were exchanged.

It was made more than apparent to me that, as far as he was concerned, this case was closed.

It is not my nature to close cases so easily. Nope! I am definitely not a case-closer.

I can't.

I won't.

And, I didn't.

Under no circumstances, was I going to shut the door on this pregnancy *case* by having an abortion. Rather, I was determined to keep that particular door wide open, and nurture and support it until the day the Lord calls me home.

I prefer to keep *cases* open until they reach an honorable completion.

Some *cases*, in fact, should remain open indefinitely. Think about that for awhile. After awhile, it should begin to make sense to you – depending on the *case*.

When Danny was born, I called his biological father to inform him of this precious baby's birth. I felt that doing so was the proper course of action, despite his obvious disinterest.

I had already mentally prepared myself for the less-than-interested response.

I do not recall his exact words in response to my news of Danny's birth - probably because they were not of a memorable nature. And unquestionably, they were *not* of a jubilant nature.

You see, jubilation does not cause a young girl to cry herself to sleep.

While still a patient in the hospital (in those days when a baby was born, mother and child stayed hospitalized much longer than is the current recommendation), a nurse assigned to my care mentioned to me that after visiting hours one evening, a fellow came by asking to see *"his baby"... my* baby. But because visiting hours were over, he was turned away.

Was it really *him*? Who knows? He never called me to say that he was coming; nor, did he call to say that he was there and was turned away.

He did show up at my house when Danny was two weeks old … just to take a look. He didn't stay. He didn't even take a seat when offered. And he showed up one more time, two years later. Again, just to take a look. And again, he did not stay.

We have not heard from him since.

More than thirty-three years have passed now with … nothing - absolutely nothing from the biological father.

I will not mention his name. It doesn't matter.

In fact, I didn't even mention his name on the birth certificate. It didn't matter.

I remember while I was in the hospital, shortly after giving birth to Danny, I was completing the paperwork regarding information that would appear on his birth certificate. The nurse assigned to my care that particular day was not only kind and compassionate, but quite insightful as well. She asked me if there was anything she could do to help me. There was.

I said, *"I'm not sure what to do about filling in the father's information on this birth certificate."* Her response to me was simply, *"Honey, you don't have to fill it in at all if you don't want to."*

I didn't want to. And, I gave Danny *my* last name.

After all, I was the one really wanting to be his parent. I was the one who chose to give him life. I was the one keeping this *case* open. I was the responsible party.

Just like his name wasn't printed on the birth certificate, you won't see the biological father's name in print on the pages of this book either.

In fact, you will not read any further mention of the biological father in my story at all.

Why not?

- Because he made no efforts to be a part of this story.
- Because he did not make his own voice heard.
- Because he did not take any responsibility whatsoever regarding Danny.
- And, because I have no information available.

Danny and I don't need to be hit over the head to realize that by the biological father's own choice, his part of this *case* continues to be closed.

And, that's okay. In fact, better than okay. Enough said.

Whether today or yesteryear, there aren't too many peers in the society of unwed pregnant teenagers. Indeed, there weren't any peers of this nature during the days of *my own* unwed teen experience. Or, at least – I had none.

Oh, there were pregnant teenagers alright. Some who I knew quite well, and some who were friends. But, they either got married before the baby was born, or they had an abortion.

So, at least in *my own* neck of the woods, there was only one in my peer group … me.

I stood alone.

I feel the need to continue to remind you that this very personal story of my own dealings with unwed teen pregnancy took place back in the 1970s – a time quite unlike the present day, where unwed teen pregnancies are much more commonplace, and much more *accepted*.

In the 1970s, typically, the unwed pregnant teen was the only peer in her group.

Single.

Solitary.

Lonely.

Do not misunderstand. Once Danny was born, it was well worth my affiliation with self-imposed solitude.

Though the only one of my friends who was pregnant at the time, I wasn't always completely alone. I still had friends that would visit me at home, and even invite me to their homes … if their parents would allow.

It didn't seem to matter, or these parents were just oblivious, that their own daughters were not entirely innocent regarding sexual experiences. Some were quite experienced, in fact. Much more than myself. Some even got pregnant, but had abortions without their parents' knowledge. Yes folks, a young teenager can get an abortion <u>without</u> *parental consent*. Don't allow yourselves to be naive regarding the abortion laws.

The friendships I had post-pregnancy just weren't what they used to be. It just wasn't the same. I couldn't just be a kid anymore.

Who in the world was I?

Pregnant at 16

Where in the world did I fit in?

I went to summer school during my pregnancy. I did this so that I could graduate from high school one year early. I wanted to graduate early so that I could get a full-time job sooner in order to be financially responsible for my child and myself.

You see, my maternal instincts were kicking in already.

So, while my friends were off enjoying their summer at the ball park, the pool, the amusement park, or just hanging out with friends - I was driving in the fast lane toward completion of my education, and my early entrance into the worlds of adulthood and parenthood.

I remember one particularly lonely occasion that summer quite clearly, as though it happened only yesterday. This happened to be just one of many times during my teen pregnancy when I was hit hard with the reality that there were some things from which I would be left out ... not because people wanted to leave me out, but because my pregnancy wouldn't allow me to be a participant in some activities.

It was a particularly hard hit when I was unable to go to a very popular, in fact world-wide known amusement park with my cousin, Karen, and her friends who came from Michigan to stay with my parents and me for a few days.

Karen was a lot of fun and had some really cool friends. They were all very kind and gracious to me. They even invited me to come with them to the amusement park for the day.

With a heavy heart, I declined.

If I had chosen to accept their sweet invitation to join them at the amusement park, I would not have been able to join them on the roller coasters.

Instead, I would have only been able to walk around, probably quite aimlessly, and likely feeling sorry for myself, while stuffing my face with fair-like junk food, and perhaps tormenting my emotions even further by watching a live dancing show surrounded by folks in the audience around my grandparents' age.

I wasn't declining my cousin's friendship. Rather, I was avoiding the feeling of aloneness while in the midst of friends.

Dorothy, a dear friend of our family, threw me a baby shower late that summer. It meant so much to me, even the *idea* that someone would consider throwing a baby shower for *"the likes of me."* It's more than merely memorable. Specifically, it's a time that I'm certain will be forever perfectly etched in my mind.

I remember that Dorothy and I and my mother were standing at the kitchen counter in our home, preparing lunch and coffee for ourselves, when Dorothy presented her baby shower *idea* to me and my mother.

Time stood still.

Wow! A shower for me and my baby? Things were beginning to *look up*.

True friends do those sorts of things, things like helping us *look up*, and:

- Lifting us up, when we're feeling down.
- Helping us out, when we're feeling helpless.
- Loving us, when we're feeling unlovable.
- Making life worthwhile, when we're feeling worthless.
- Guiding us, when we're feeling lost.
- Showing us the bright side, when we feel surrounded by darkness.

The genuine love that was shown to me by Dorothy, the shower guests, and family members was amazing. No, *mind-blowing!*

It was especially amazing when contrasted with the folks on the other end of the spectrum who are known to have remarked that the shower and gifts were *"inappropriate"*, given my *"situation."*

I quit going to church when the awareness of my pregnancy could not be hidden any longer.

My pre-pregnancy clothing didn't fit anymore. My waistline became non-existent rapidly. So, it was necessary for me to begin wearing maternity clothes very early on in my pregnancy.

And of course, *word got around* that I was expecting, and I was not prepared emotionally to deal with responses from others regarding my *condition* - whether nice or not-so-nice.

Remember, I was *only sixteen*. Only sixteen, in an adult situation.

I didn't quit going to church because I felt like I wouldn't be accepted. I quit going because I was ashamed and embarrassed no matter how much people would tell me that I was welcome there.

Beyond a shadow of a doubt, I knew that I would stand out more than just like a sore thumb.

And, though there were many genuinely caring folks who loved me even with all my shortcomings, and maybe loved me even a little more given my circumstances - I was quite aware that there might be a few negative whispers that included my name, shameful fingers being pointed in my direction, and fiery darts piercing my heart by those who were convinced that my *unconcealed* sins were far worse than their own *concealed* sins.

I promptly recognized however, that there were a great many more members of the congregation who possessed genuinely caring hearts than those who may have been hardhearted.

As a matter of fact, I cannot bring to mind any *whispers, fingers,* or *darts*.

That's not to say there weren't any – but, even if there were … my own awareness of such *was* and *is* non-existent.

A few teens from my Sunday school class would call me on the telephone, or write kind letters of encouragement to me, or send sweet messages to me through my mom who attended church regularly.

One of the kind letters, from Anna Beth (whom I mentioned earlier in this text), included the words, *"I love you."*

It still makes me cry - *tears of joyfulness.*

And a few folks older than me, most around my mom and dad's age, even dropped by the house on occasion … just to visit with me.

Me! I was important to them, as evidenced by their sincere confirmation of love toward me, as well as their selfless acts of kindness.

You know how some things just come to mind so much more often than others? Well, I happen to have a clear recollection of a noteworthy occurrence while I was pregnant, and still choosing to stay home from church for reasons that I've already mentioned.

I was home alone.

I believe my mom had just stepped out for a few minutes to stop by the grocery store, when I heard the doorbell ring. It was somebody from church.

As I peeked out the window, and before making the decision to go ahead and answer the door, I remember thinking, *"Great! (sarcasm) Somebody from church! And, I'm here alone. This is going to be awkward."*

I had no idea what to expect when I apprehensively answered that door. I figured, *"Guess it's time I finally face the music,"* so to speak.

This was my very first visit from somebody from church (other than my mom and dad's good friends, Dorothy and Frank, and their three children – who were also teenagers, by the way).

This kind visitor's name was Mrs. Vernier. Back in those days, anyone who was considered to be your elder was *always* addressed as either *Mr., Miss, or Mrs.* preceding their last name. It was considered disrespectful to call an elder by their first name, unless he or she was a close friend of the family, in which case you were allowed to add a respectful *Aunt* or *Uncle* before stating their first name, but only if by prior approval which involved a consult with your parents.

Nevertheless, when I answered the door and greeted Mrs. Vernier with an artificial smile that I worked hard to muster up, I immediately told her, *"My mom's not home right now."* To my surprise, she promptly responded, *"I didn't come to see your mom. I came to see you."*

What?

She came to see me?

I was puzzled, to say the least. Why would she want to see me?

And how in the world was I supposed to hold a conversation with someone my mom's age, especially with this obvious big belly of mine which I felt was screaming – *"Yep, one of those wild teenagers houses this pregnant belly."*

I was nervous.

My nervousness, I'm sure, was due to my certainty that we were nothing less than worlds apart.

In no time at all however, Mrs. Vernier proved my *"worlds apart"* theory incorrect. Her pleasant manner and evidence of authentic ease in the art of conversation even with a teenager – a teenager like me – an unwed, pregnant teenager – took a firm hold of my uneasiness and threw it right out the window.

Her undeniable proof of genuine love for me, no matter the situation I currently found myself in, demonstrated to me that we weren't worlds apart at all. Nope. We shared the same world. We shared the same love for children. In fact, we shared a lot of the same thoughts and ideas. We certainly shared the same love for God. We even shared the same love for each other. And, we even learned a lot about each other.

We had a good time. It turned out to be quite an enlightening and delightfully memorable occasion.

The nice, long chat we enjoyed that afternoon was not about anything in particular.

It turned out to be an unexpected but extraordinary visit between two ladies only one generation apart, not too much unlike a visit that you might have with any of your good friends who might just take a notion to pop in on you on any given day and, just because they genuinely care about you.

She did not make me feel guilty.

She did not make me feel ashamed.

She did not carry any darts in her pocket that might pierce my heart.

The only thing she carried with her was the unconditional love in her heart that she so graciously shared with me. Oh, she did carry one more thing … a present for my baby.

I don't recall what the present was. It might have been a baby blanket or something. It's the thought that counts, right? And, she was certainly thoughtful.

But, the best present of all that afternoon, was the sincere lovingkindness and friendship that was shown to me in a manner that caught me off guard, but was enormously welcomed and will be remembered forever – lovingly.

Although I did not attend church for the remainder of my pregnancy, my mom and I would have daily Bible studies together.

It was a mutual decision to do this. I desperately wanted to experience these one-on-one Bible studies, and to get back in step with my walk with Jesus. And my mom encouraged this. She was my cheerleader.

When we finished one study, I could hardly wait until the next day when we'd sit at the kitchen table, or in the living room, or even in my bedroom, and do it all over again. I even asked my mom to tell me again the Bible stories that I should have paid more attention to when I was younger. I simply could not remember most of them.

When I was a young child in Sunday school, I was just a kid like many others whose focusing abilities were far from top notch. Mine just might have been a little further from that notch than others.

But, I had a new determination during the summer of 1974 to pay very close attention to my newest Bible teacher – my dear mother.

That summer of my teenage pregnancy was the year that I turned my life back over to Christ - forever.

My mom became my best friend.

My mom was my peer.

I was in her *group*.

She was the one I wanted to be more like. I looked up to her. She was my hero. Still is!

We shopped together, went out to lunch together, played board games together, went for walks together, watched television shows together, went to drive-in movies together, had our Bible studies daily together, and laughed out loud together - a lot. Delightful and often uncontrollable laughter.

That's what best friends do.

My best friend - my mom - was an ever-present listening ear, and even just a comforting presence when I didn't want to talk at all. She was there for me. Always.

She was my emotional uplifter. And she was so good at it, you'd think she'd taken a course wherein she received the highest degree possible in emotional uplifting. But, no - she was just innately an expert.

What a gift!

What a blessing!

As you surely must be able to imagine, my mom's career in emotional uplifting, especially during my pregnancy and the early years of Danny's life, was at times a twenty-four hour a day job. Better yet, let us say that she was *on call* twenty-four hours a day.

She was there to answer all of my *fear of the unknown* questions, and to guide and direct me in the way only a loving, godly mother can do. And what an outstanding job she did!

She was there when I asked these questions (among others):
- How is this pregnancy going to change my life?
- How is this baby going to change my life?
- How can Jesus still love a sinner like me?
- How can I know for certain that I am a Christian?
- How do I take care of this baby?
- Will anyone want to marry me?
- How and when do I tell my baby he was conceived out of wedlock?
- How am I going to be able to support my baby on my own?
- Will I ever be able to do fun things again with my friends without feeling guilty about leaving my baby with a babysitter (which was always my parents, by the way)?
- Will the kids at church accept me back into the youth group after I give birth? After all, I'll still be *youthful.*
- How do I handle or respond to people who gossip about me?
- Why do people look down on me for giving life, but say nothing about the girl who ended her baby's life through abortion?
- Why are there some people who don't feel comfortable celebrating my baby's birth? After all, I'm excited about my baby, and proud of him, and want to show him off.
- What if there's something physically or mentally wrong with my baby? Is it my fault?
- What does it feel like to give birth?

- Will you stay with me while I'm in labor with my baby? I didn't want to be alone. It seemed incredibly scary to me.
- Why do some people keep telling me that I should give my baby up for adoption?
- Why do some people avoid me now?
- Will these stretch marks ever go away?
- Does Jesus forgive me?

At all times, my mom was there for me.

At all times, she uplifted me.

And at all times, she affectionately and tenderly imparted her remarkable wisdom to my sometimes tough-to-answer questions.

CHAPTER SIX

TEEN MOTHERHOOD

*"Behold, children are a heritage from the Lord,
The fruit of the womb is a reward."
Psalm 127: 3*

It was nearly 3:00 p.m.

The sun was shining, a comfortable breeze was blowing, and the leaves on the two maple trees on our lush front lawn had already changed from gorgeous greens to brilliant shades of yellows, oranges, and reds.

We had all the windows and doors open in our midwestern home purposefully to enjoy the cool breezes flowing through the screens and onto our exposed skin.

My mom and dad and I were sitting at the kitchen table enjoying this gorgeous day and the company of one another when … my labor began.

This was it.

It was really happening.

And, it was really scary.

Again, I feel compelled to remind you that I was only sixteen. *Only sixteen!*

Prior to the pregnancy and birthing process, my two biggest fears were darkness and needles. But now, I was coming face to face with labor and childbirth. This is stuff that adults are supposed to be prepared for, not me ... not a teenager.

Often, I think back about when my own children were just sixteen years old. They were just kids. They were still *my babies*.

I was just a baby myself, but in an instant I would be transformed into a mother. In just a few short hours, I would be holding my own little baby in my arms - at long last. Or, did the past nine months just fly by?

I didn't know if I was going to have a little boy or a little girl. Remember, things have changed tremendously over the past thirty-five years.

Back then, the sex of the baby was a surprise - at the very moment of birth. At ... not before.

I didn't care whether my child was male or female, as long as he or she was healthy.

Whether my child was completely healthy or not was always weighing very heavily on my mind during my pregnancy. In secret, and daily, I would pray - no, plead - with the Lord to *"Please, please give me a perfectly healthy child."*

Looking back, I think the reason I carried this heavy weight was three-fold.

- First, I felt that my young age might be a negative factor on the health of this child.
- Second, I thought my being given an unhealthy baby would be my punishment to fit my *crime*.
- Third and probably foremost, I was so concerned that if my baby required any extra care, my poor parents would be forced to share in that burden – magnifying my already guilty complex.

So my prayers for a healthy child continued … day and night.

Now the time had come. I would find out in just a few short hours both the sex and the health of my child.

I thought that I was prepared for what was to come - the labor. I was not.

I thought you were supposed to be able to rest between the contractions. I did not.

I thought I'd be able to handle this on my own. I could not. I would not. And, I did not.

The contractions began with a bang. One big bang right on top of another.

Epidurals were not commonplace at that time. In fact, I'm not even really sure if they were *in* place at all in 1974.

In any case, an epidural was nothing I had ever heard of at that time.

Even if it was available, it was not something that was offered to me.

So, I endured the labor, but not alone.

My mom was at my side, holding my hand, encouraging me, and all the while looking at me with those distinctive *"mom eyes."* Once again and true to form, my mother's remarkable nature was shining through - brilliantly!

I don't think she ever let go of my hand. Moms are like that. Most importantly however, she held my heart. Still does!

At 7:04 p.m., I gave birth to a son - Danny – eight pounds, two ounces, twenty-one inches long, and the cutest baby I had ever seen in my life. Really! And, he was mine. All mine. At least, that's what I remember thinking that glorious, incredible, amazing moment in time.

Soon thereafter I also came to the realization that God not only blessed me with Danny, but that He entrusted me with his care. Me!

You could say I gave birth to two people on October 4, 1974. I didn't realize it immediately, but at the moment of Danny's birth I also gave birth to a new *me*.

Instinctively, I took on the role of *Mommy*. In my mind, I carried my whole *mommy check list:*

- Does he have all his fingers and toes?
- Does he have an intact sucking reflex?
- Is he remembering to breathe while asleep?
- Is he going to be all right physically?
- Is he going to be all right emotionally?
- Is he hungry?
- Is he thirsty?
- Is he cold?
- Is he hot?
- Is his diaper wet or dirty?
- Is he happy?
- Is he sad?
- Do those nurses really know what my baby needs?
- Does he know I'm his mommy?
- Am I doing everything right?
- Are they really going to let me take this tiny little creature out of the hospital?

And …

- I hope he loves me.

Motherhood was better than I could have hoped or dreamed. Yep – even at sixteen.

I was in love with my precious little baby boy. Love that truly began from the time my mom uttered the word *"pregnant"* to me on that bittersweet ride home from high school months earlier.

I went back to school. The students were gracious enough - to my face. Truth be known, they were probably more curious than anything else.

I had a best friend, Letha, who stuck by me through thick and thin. She had attended my baby shower and brought me a beautiful soft white blanket for my precious Danny. I later found out that she skipped eating lunch many times just so that she could save her lunch money to purchase the white blanket for Danny. To this day, her generosity and selflessness brings tears to my eyes. What a friend!

I believe that most of the teachers just *put up* with me. Like I was so hard to *put up* with! Sheesh! They didn't know the real me from Adam. And, it was quite clear that getting to know me was not an opportunity they wished to pursue.

However, I do feel compelled to gratefully acknowledge two of my high school teachers. They went out of their way to make me understand that my life was not a fiasco but, rather – that my life had significance.

They were both born again Christians. They assisted me in taking some high school classes at home during the last few months of my pregnancy and for a short while thereafter.

Better yet, they got to know me. The *real Lori*. And they demonstrated a genuine interest in me, despite my imperfections. They found the good in me, and taught me how to appreciate the good, to build on that goodness, and to rise above my weaknesses.

In other words, their respect for me as a person helped me to overcome my weaknesses and made me stronger in so many ways.

Ultimately, isn't that what teachers are supposed to do?

They didn't just *do* their job – they did an *extraordinary* job.

I went back to church. It was a little unnerving at first. I knew that everyone there was aware of my *situation*. I was still very much a *kid* myself, but happened to be a *kid* leaving her own *kid* in the nursery.

Pregnant at 16

Without doubt, I was alone in that category.

I wondered how the nursery workers would react upon my arrival with Danny. I was so relieved when it was our family friend, Dorothy, who met me at the nursery door, her arms outstretched for me *and* Danny. She had the biggest smile on her face, and her welcoming arms made my heart melt.

You remember Dorothy. She's the one who threw my baby shower.

Her manner of greeting seemed to spread like wildfire among other members of the congregation. She took Danny from my arms and showed him off like he was a prince.

He *was* a prince. *My* prince.

Yes, I felt like I was being welcomed home. Genuinely and warmly welcomed. Like the Scripture says, *"I was glad when they said unto me – Let us go into the House of the Lord."* I was thrilled to be back *home*.

Next was Sunday school. What would the *welcome* be like there?

I'd be lying if I said it wasn't at all awkward. It *was* awkward. Awkward for me *and* equally as awkward, I'm sure, for the other *kids* in my class.

I feel the need to continue to remind you that we were *all* just *kids*.

The awkwardness didn't last long though. Although I was not greeted with the same enthusiasm I experienced when leaving Danny in the nursery - the other *kids* smiled at me, talked to me, asked me if I had any pictures of Danny, and some even walked to the nursery with me after Sunday School so that they could meet Danny.

I was beaming with pride. Danny was so cute, and he was mine. Hey – the *kids* even asked me if I wanted to join them after the evening church service at one of their homes for singing, snacks, and fellowship. With a very glad heart, I said, *"Sure."*

It was a very good day.

It's very important to me that I mention one more fellow at church by name. Gilbert Elliott. He was a very nice older gentleman who always stood at the back of the Church greeting folks upon their arrival and shaking hands and giving heart-felt hugs prior to their departure.

Before I got pregnant with Danny, Mr. Elliott always shook my hand on Sunday mornings and Sunday evenings, and he always called me his *girlfriend*. He was a very sweet man, and *"girlfriend"* was just his innocent term of endearment for me.

When I saw Mr. Elliott at church for the first time since Danny's birth – I hadn't seen Mr. Elliott in months, by the way – he greeted me again, with the same enthusiasm as always, as if nothing at all had changed.

Yes – as if we *hadn't missed a lick,* except that *this time* he pulled me a little closer and softly uttered these unforgettable words, *"Lori, you're still my girlfriend"*.

How overwhelmingly awesome is that! Honestly, tears well up every time I recall that precious moment.

I was more than impressed by and grateful for the genuine love that was shown toward me by so many people whose hearts were obviously filled with the love of God.

So impressed was I, in fact, that their love caused me to gain a significant foothold on the bridge that carried me from *troubled waters* to *rivers of peace with God.*

I was filled with a renewed inner desire to become significantly more involved in church and to take a lifelong closer walk with Jesus Christ.

One night when I and a group of my friends went bowling, we ran into and ultimately became friends with a group of teenagers as well as younger adults in their early twenties who were obviously on fire for the Lord.

They were at the bowling alley handing out tracts (Christian mini-pamphlets explaining the way of salvation through Jesus

Christ) and talking to other teenagers like myself about the Lord Jesus and how to *get saved.*

I was already a Christian. I had already asked the Lord into my heart as a young child. But, their M.O. (method of operation) intrigued me because I had already decided during my pregnancy that I was no longer going to be quiet about the things of the Lord.

Yes - I was determined that I was finally and at long last going to let my voice be heard, and tell others about the saving grace of Jesus.

These young folks had quite a catchy slogan on the subject of getting saved. It was *"Get Smart! Get Saved!"* At that time, they called themselves the *"Forever Family."* I've checked – and they're still around. But apparently now there are only a few hundred of them across the nation, and as far as I know, they have since changed their *name.*

It is my understanding that the reason for the name change *was* due to the *"Forever Family"* sounding too much like a hippie group living in a commune. I am convinced as well that they deemed the name change a necessity in order to be assured that there would be no misconception regarding any connection to another infamous family – e.g., *"Charlie's"* family.

In any case, in the 1970s, there were thousands of members of this *"Forever Family."* And, it is my belief that they simply chose the word *family* because they were all a part of the big *family of God.* And, most of the members were new to the whole idea of getting saved and following Jesus. So, the *family* name was truly and simply an innocent choice of words.

Don't read anything more into it, because it's nothing more than that.

I was more than excited about the *Forever Family* and about attending their weekly Bible studies in someone's home.

I told my Mom and Dad all about it.

They were a little more than skeptical. Understandably.

So, I invited my dad and a friend of his to come to one of our Bible studies, asking the other members first if they minded if some folks from the *older generation* attended a meeting or two.

They didn't mind at all.

My dad, in particular, was interested in finding out for himself just what in the world these young people were all about. I am sure his greatest concern was, *"Is Lori getting herself involved with some kind of cult?"*

That was a reasonable concern.

He likely was even thinking - *"Great! First, the pregnancy. Now, this."* And, *"Is my youngest daughter now going to be living in some kind of hippie commune?"*

For those of you a generation or two behind me, hippie communes were quite common back then.

The *Forever Family* Bible study that my dad and his friend attended, along with me and my friend, Letha, went quite well. And, I'm pretty sure my dad and his friend were more pleased than they originally thought they might be.

One of the things that the *Forever Family* strongly encouraged was Scripture memorization. In fact, there were quite a number of verses that folks in the group were encouraged to memorize. Most of the verses had to do with the plan of salvation.

Once you memorized these particular verses (as I recall, there were a total of twenty), you earned a button to wear that bore their slogan, *"Get Smart! Get Saved!"*

During the meeting, my dad and his friend made it known that they would each like to have one of those buttons for themselves. Well, the leader of the Bible study said, *"You'll have to earn it. You have to memorize the verses first."*

After inquiring further, my dad and his buddy said that they would like to try to earn their buttons that very night. Some of the members of the *Forever Family* just giggled quietly amongst themselves. I'm certain they were thinking, *"Yeah, right – like these two old guys are gonna recite all twenty of the verses tonight – without error."*

Well … they did! Without cheating. And, error-free.

I was so proud. And, they each proudly wore their *"Get Smart! – Get Saved!"* buttons home that evening. I guess that made them members of the *family* too. Although – technically, they were *already* members of the *family* … the *family of God*.

So encouraged was I by my father's Bible verse knowledge, and well as delighted by his willingness to attend the meeting with me, that I challenged myself to be more like him. He was my role model. Still is!

Challenge! That was it! I was going to challenge myself to be more of what God wanted me to be. And, I continue to this day to work hard at that.

From time to time though, I find myself lost in the thought, *"You've still got a long way to go, Lori."*

Nonetheless, I still had to deal with the *challenge* of unwed, teenage motherhood. That produced an even bigger mountain to climb. And, what a gargantuan mountain it was!

The climb could be awfully exhausting at times, physically as well as mentally. Especially when you're *only sixteen!*

One of the biggest challenges of being an unwed teenage mother is that you don't have anyone to share your parenting role with.

You are *it*.

Just you.

Alone.

In my particular case however, I did have my parents – with whom Danny and I continued to reside - to guide me regarding the *ins and outs* of parenthood.

And of course, this meant that Danny and I were doubly blessed because his *Grandma and Grandpa Ghiata* were ever-present sources of love, hope, encouragement, guidance, and uplifting.

Indeed, my parents/Danny's grandparents deserve immeasurable admiration for their perpetual and much appreciated assistance in our *distinctive* situation.

Nonetheless, Danny was without a father. Yes, you read that right. No daddy. So, this made me *both* mom *and* dad.

That was a real trick sometimes because although the *mom* role I had taken on (the nurturing/emotional role) came with a rather intuitive knack, the *dad* role was initially unfamiliar territory for me.

This required a behavior that I had never before learned to demonstrate.

Certainly, it was not a role that I instinctively knew how to play.

So, I thought it was important to also take on a role incorporating a somewhat strict performance – like many fathers innately do.

Perhaps the character I played was a little *over the top* at times – but, I just wanted to make sure that my performance as both mother *and* father was that of an award-winning nature.

My dad would sometimes say, *"You run a tight ship, Lori."*

You see, my father was a Captain on a ship – a cement freighter on the Great Lakes - so *"running a tight ship"* was something with which he was very familiar.

And, it's my understanding and belief that if you want your *ship* to run smoothly and according to knowledge about what works and what doesn't work, *tight ships* are a pretty good example to follow.

I didn't necessarily want to run the tightest ship around, but I wanted to run one that was at least respectable. I guess I wanted desperately to be *mom extraordinaire.*

Clearly, my goal was to be the single mom to be admired for her extraordinary abilities to handle a not-so-perfect situation in such a way that would hopefully cause onlookers to remark, *"She's doing an outstanding parenting job, given her unusual circumstances!"*

I was determined to give a *stand out* performance in my dual role as a momma *and* a daddy, particularly to those that said, *"She'll never make it."* and, *"Her poor little boy doesn't stand a chance having an unwed teenage mother."*

Without a doubt, I was *going to show them.*

I was going to show them that, *"Yes, I can do it, and I'll do an exceptional job."*

Needless to say, the task set before me (or, better said – the task I set before myself) was a whopping big task. But, I was filled with just as whopping a determination that I would immerse myself daily in accomplishing my task with flying colors.

After all, I had a lot of proving to do.

I had something to prove to others, something to prove to myself, and most importantly, something to prove to Danny, because I loved him so much, and more than anything else on this earth.

What was I thinking? I didn't have to do this completely on my own.

No!

I finally had to convince myself to *wake up and smell the coffee.* Good grief! Talk about *not being able to see the forest for the trees.*

True – Danny did not have a daddy living in our home. But, he *did* have Grandma and Grandpa Ghiata… living in the same house.

And, how cool is that!

My mom and dad are like the grandma and grandpa you read about in the storybooks. Oh, yes! They are *that* special to their grandkids, and to *all* of us who love them, for that matter.

The *storybook-ness* of it all, however, had its *lessons to be learned* chapters as well. And I must say that I am more than blessed to have had the remarkable and humbling opportunity to learn the fine points of parenthood from some of the most excellent parents ever created.

I had a *bonus* too, although I didn't realize the bonus until many years later when Danny and his wife, Erin, blessed Joe and myself with our first grandchild – Lindsey Brooke Bowser on May 13, 2003.

Yes, living with my parents for the first three years of Danny's life afforded me the additional benefit of learning the treasured art of grandparenting from role model grandparents – Don and Thais Ghiata.

Without question, there were some storybook qualities to my life at that time. But, let's not forget that my teenage life was far from being a fairy tale experience.

Once again, and probably not for the last time, I am going to remind you … I was *only sixteen!*

Even though I was a mother – a mother that would have liked to have won the *mom of the year award* if there ever was one - I was still a teenager.

And, a foremost thought that seems to incessantly reside in the mind of every sixteen year old girl is this: Dating.

More *challenges!*

- Some guys don't want to date someone who has a child out of wedlock.
- Some guys *want* to date you because they think you're *easy* because you've had a child out of wedlock.
- You want to make certain that the guy you're dating likes children – especially *your* child.
- You aren't always available to date, because you have responsibilities regarding your child. And, your child comes first.
- Some guys take offense that your child comes first.
- So, you *write off* the guy who takes offense.

- Some guys *spoil your child* only because they want to impress you, but you find out later that their lavish gifts and attention given to your child weren't at all sincere.
- And, yeah – you might not look quite so *hot* in that bikini anymore due to the pregnancy-induced stretch marks. (Wear a one-piece bathing suit? Are you kidding me? I might *be* somebody's momma, but I sure ain't gonna sport one of those *momma* swimsuits.)

It's been said, *"When the going gets tough, the tough get going."*

My personal *"going"* experiences, especially when compared with the *"goings"* other kids my own age, certainly caused me to *toughen up*. And admittedly, many of my own *"tough goings"* were self-induced.

Nonetheless, good friends can help lighten the load. In fact, friendships are yet another essential feature in a teenager's life. And, every teenager needs at least a few really good friends who they can count on to be there – *especially* when the going gets tough. The problem is ... *some* of the parents of *some* of your friends.

- Some of your friends' parents have decided that they no longer want their kids to be friends with you because you might be a bad influence. In these parents' minds, you have now become the dreaded *bad girl*.
- Their daughter might get pregnant because you got pregnant. (What? ... I might not be the brightest crayon in the box, but I'm pretty sure it doesn't work that way.)

I did have some of those *stick to ya like glue* girlfriends, though. They *toughed it out* right along with me.

For that, dear friends, I am forever grateful.

You know who you are.

It's also worth mentioning that many of my *guy* friends demonstrated an unanticipated, but well-received, absolute maturity regarding my whole *situation* as well. These fellas proved to be just good ole boys who wanted nothing more than to carry on with the simple friendships we had always enjoyed … *pre-Danny*. How refreshing!

These guys and gals didn't simply *pick up where we left off*. Nope. They never *left* in the first place.

When all's said and done, you really *do* know who your *real* friends are when the glue that binds you together is nothing less than *super*.

CHAPTER SEVEN
TELLING MY KIDS

*"Confess your trespasses to one another,
And pray for one another, that you may be healed.
The effective, fervent prayer of a righteous man avails much."
James 5: 16*

Where did we get the idea that our children are supposed to think that we've never done anything wrong? Do we really expect them to believe …

- That we never talked out of turn? (Yes, you did.)
- That we never lied to our parents? (You know there are those times when you've said, *"not me"*, when in fact it was no one *but* you.)
- That we never cheated on a test? (Remember, I was the *not-so-smart kid* who positioned herself strategically in the classroom on *verbal quiz day*.)
- That we never skipped school? (Really? Was your name not on the absentee report on *Senior Skip Day* in high school?)
- And, that we never *fell down*, and had to pick ourselves up again, by our bootstraps?

Furthermore, there were those times when we couldn't even find our boots, let alone the straps to grab whereby we could pull ourselves up out of whatever mess we'd gotten ourselves into.

Even more frustrating – once the boots and their straps had been found, the boots didn't fit quite right.

Maybe they were too big, and we just needed to allow maturity to develop allowing for the time to grow into them, as well as working hard to gain the needed strength to tighten our grip.

Once those big shoes begin to fit a little more snugly, it is then that you are able to put one foot in front of the other and take one step at a time.

I am convinced that my parents were as close to perfect role models for parenthood (and grandparenthood, for that matter) as one can get. I wanted to be like them. So, I tried to follow their *perfect-in-my-eyes* examples.

For the record, this is an ongoing aspiration … to be more like my mom and dad.

Yes, I have fallen from time to time; but, my mom and dad are successful trainers in effectively teaching folks to search for and find their own boots, take hold of the bootstraps, and pick one's self up again and with a firmer grip each time.

Nevertheless, when my own children became teenagers, I am embarrassed now to admit that on a relatively routine basis a thought that seemed to preoccupy my mind was this, *"So much for being a role model for my own kids."*

No. It didn't simply preoccupy my mind. Instead, it was more like that thought was impersonating a prison guard keeping his ever-watchful eye on his captive.

What in the world was I doing?

Undeniably, I was being held prisoner by my own harshly critical thought processes. I seemed to be fixated on self-defeat.

I wondered how long I would be locked in this *self-destructive* cell? How long would I be *"doing time"*? Was it a *"life sentence"*?

You see, during each of my children's journeys through adolescence, that miserable DVD player in my mind would quickly rewind back to my own personal experiences with adolescent struggles and insecurities.

And quite self-destructively, I kept *re-viewing* my past poor judgments.

Although I am very proud of the way my own children handled the potentially turbulent teenage years, I was still very much ashamed of the way I handled my own.

It was no secret to my children that Danny was born out of wedlock to me when I was still a teenager. They seemed to handle that information quite maturely, understandingly, lovingly, and without difficulty.

But for me, I was still embarrassed, and maybe even a little jealous because, as compared with my own teen experiences, my kids – most of the time – had *the times of their lives* during their teen years.

That was something that I, for the most part, had missed out on.

The jealousy was just a *miniature* part of my thought processes, though. More predominant was the chronic torment to my inner self that my *past* might not only embarrass my children, but might not leave me any room for instilling in my own children proper morals and godly behaviors.

After all I thought, it had well been established and beyond a reasonable doubt that I was guilty of committing the offense for which I was charged.

Though I was trapped in self-induced solitary confinement, all measurable evidence validates my notion that I wasn't at all destroying my children's self-images. My three kids, though different as night and day, gave the impression of being quite self-assured.

It was reasonably apparent that they were not at all bothered by my *real* image. As a matter of fact, they always gave me the feeling that they loved me just as I was - even with all my imperfections, blunders, mistakes, weaknesses, and shortcomings.

Let me take even one step further out on this limb and say that I believe it is *because* of my mistakes, *because* of my picking myself up by my bootstraps, and *because* of my honesty with my kids that they have become upstanding, caring, and respected adults.

Unquestionably, and to my indescribable delight, my teenage history did not *generate* a negative influence to this *next generation* of mine.

In other words, I didn't pass on a *bad gene* to my kids.

Forget the *"apple and the tree"* theory.

My *apples* (namely – Danny, Shannon, and Shelby) fell in three very different locations, but in all three cases – very far from *this tree* (me) … well – the *old* me.

Whereas, regarding the *new* me, please afford me this opportunity to *toot my own horn* by declaring that I'm convinced I imparted to my own kids a number of good quality characteristics of which I am swollen with pride.

I'm not knocking the value of psychology, but I would emphatically disagree with anyone who declares that *all* children of unwed mothers are destined to a life of poverty, decreased mental abilities, and *passing the buck* to their own children and grandchildren.

My children are just fine. Thank you very much.

Why?

I'm persuaded to think that maybe, just maybe it's because I learned from my own mistakes and worked feverishly to make certain that my kids didn't follow in their momma's wayward footsteps … you know - those footsteps that veered off the straight and narrow course.

I am not at all suggesting that my own children didn't step out of line at one time or another.

Pregnant at 16

Nope. I know all too well that most kids, especially teenagers, have an instinctively powerful curiosity about the crooked paths of life as opposed to the straight ones.

After all, society encourages all of us to think outside the box, whatever our age, and even to take that giant leap outside the box. And teenagers, especially teenagers, will give in to their inquisitive instincts by taking at least a mini excursion (possibly, even several such excursions) along a trail daringly marked *proceed with caution* at the trail's head.

C'mon. Is it not common knowledge that teenagers quite often give in to *the dare*?

Picture this – you've got the *dare* dude sitting on the left shoulder of the teenager, and the *been there/done that/don't do it* dude sitting on the teen's right shoulder. Though both might articulate very convincing arguments for their case, which character do you think is going to win that debate?

If you're in touch with teenagers at all, or even if your familiarity with teenagers is only that you once were one, you know that very often it's the *dare* dude who reigns triumphant.

In fact, the *dare* dude presents an even more convincing argument to the teenager if he transforms into … the *double dare* dude.

Please don't tell me you're sitting there wondering how in the world the *double dare* dude is so often victorious when up against the *been there/done that/don't do it* dude.

But in the off chance that you are questioning the reason for the repeated successes of the *dare* dude … apparently, it's because he embodies an influential nature of such enormity that it persuades teenagers to believe that his way of life is more fun and exciting.

Much more fun, and *much* more exciting.

But, it is only much later that the inquiring minds of teenagers come to realize that the *dare* dude's roads have the very real potential of turning into toll roads.

In other words, there's often a high price to be paid when passing through those subdivisions of life wherein we test the waters (or, trails) of trial and error. And, some roads are even more costly than others.

Regrettably, as a teenager, I had traveled too many *dead-end* trails and tested too many *drowning* waters.

Those *dead-end* trails led only to precious years wasted.

And, the *drowning* waters were suffocating.

All high prices I've paid for my own teenage recklessness.

After thirty-five years of quiet introspection, it became more than apparent to me that I was the only one in my immediate family that was at all disturbed by the complex details of my past wayward history.

All at once, it seemed, I realized that my reflection of self followed more along the lines of scrutiny, followed by despair, and then dysfunctionality.

That had to be changed!

Change! That was the ticket! Why hadn't I considered this solution to my predicament forever and a day ago?

I would simply change my opinion of myself by allowing myself to come to the realization that I had learned some valuable lessons from my own teenage history.

Costly lessons, yes. But, oh – so priceless, once I realized how my *lessons learned* had the potential of positively impacting the precious lives of the younger generation. Hey – maybe even older generations.

CHAPTER EIGHT
TELLING MY ADULT FRIENDS

"Judge not, that you be not judged.
For with what judgment you judge, you will be judged;
And with the measure you use, it will be measured back to you.
And, why do you look at the speck in your brother's eye,
But do not consider the plank in your own eye?
Or, how can you say to your brother,
'Let me remove the speck from your eye';
And look, a plank is in your own eye?
Hypocrite! First remove the plank from your own eye,
And then you will see clearly to remove the speck from your
brother's eye." – Matthew 7: 1-5

Telling my adult friends and acquaintances that I was an unwed teen mother ranks right up there with ... with ... well, with *nothing*.

Honestly, I cannot think of much else in my life thus far that has made me feel more uncomfortable. Indeed, verbal disclosure of my wayward teen years has been my biggest personal obstacle to overcome.

Isn't that something? It seems at times that the toughest part of my story has been the panic associated with the horror of having to repeat my story – one more painful time after another.

Not unlike many folks, when there's the possibility that I might have to endure pain, whether physical or emotional, I avoid it.

So, that's what I routinely did over the course of the past thirty-five years. I avoided my own emotional pain by dodging situations wherein I might be forced to share my story with others.

I believed that sharing my story would only initiate having to answer tough questions, which would bring about even more unwanted pain.

And then of course, there was the very real possibility that sharing my story would have that domino effect, e.g., having others share my story with even more folks, likely leading to even more questions, and thus even more pain.

More curious people.

More tough questions.

More emotional pain.

I'm not crazy about curious people, because I'm not fond of tough questions. And, I'm even less fond of emotional pain, at least not when it pertains to my personal life.

One of the most difficult times on the obstacle course that I call my life occurs when someone I'm hanging out with at that particular moment sees an unwed pregnant teenager and utters under her breath, but to me (unaware of my history, of course), and with all the negativity that she can seem to muster, questions such as:

- "What was she thinking?"
- Or, "Where were her parents?"
- Or, "Doesn't she know anything about birth control?"
- Or, "That poor unborn child's life is going to be a nightmare."
- Or, "Why didn't she have an abortion?"
- Or, "I hope she puts that baby up for adoption, and gives it to some family that really wants to have a baby, but can't."

- Or, "That girl has ruined the rest of her life."
- Or, "No man is ever going to want to marry her."

The list goes on. And yes, I have heard them all, and more.

Comments like those were the driving force causing me to keep my skeletons locked up, and my lips tightly sealed. Sheltered from opposition and hostility, for good!

Until now.

Now, I'm telling everyone. What a switch!

I compare the *switch* to a light switch in my home, except that this particular light switch is not attached to a solid wall. Rather, this *switch* is attached to the wall of my heart.

My *switch* was always kept in the *off* position with purposeful determination.

I had resolved to keep others *in the dark* regarding the *"Lori chronicles."*

And, I felt quite safe in my own personal darkness. Undeniably, I was unwavering in my resolution to keep my personal history private, and to keep others *in the dark*.

I had no intention of flipping the switch that would turn my private concerns into public knowledge.

Not only did I refuse to shed light on my very private memoirs with others, but I became lovingly accustomed to the feeling of *normalcy* by dimming my own memories as well.

Here's the *switch:*

- What was once dark, is now light.
- What was once unclear, is now clear.
- What was once a mystery, is now exposed.
- What was once black, is now white.
- What was once a closed book, is now open.

Never in my wildest dreams would I have ever thought I would finally get to this place. But, I *am* here. And, what a wonderful place it is. My fear of the unknown was unwarranted.

I carry within myself a renewed spirit, a purpose, and a plan. My life - even with its imperfections, shortcomings, weaknesses, and past failures - has a purpose.

There really *is* a reason I'm here.

In the past and up until now, self-preservation was *the* significant driving force in my secrecy regarding my unwed, teen pregnancy.

But, shame on me!

Shame on me for keeping so quiet for the greater part of the last thirty-five years – thirty-five long, quiet years of my life that could have *instead* been spent sharing my story purposefully to help others, and thereby glorifying Jesus' name.

Time flies! The past thirty-five years seem to have passed in a flash/in the blink of an eye.

When I was a little girl, I can recall routinely hearing the older generation frequently utter, *"Life is so short."* They were right. Now that I am *one of them*, I realize with intense clarity the truth in that statement.

If you are not *one of them* yet, you soon will be … tomorrow.

And when you hold onto something heartrending, refusing to let it out and let it go - like I did for so many years - eventually what used to be just a twinge or tenderness is ultimately going to fester into throbbing pain followed by unrelenting anguish.

I am disappointed in my former self – the self that avoided sharing my story for so many years.

On the brighter side, I am finally – and at long last - satisfied with my present-day self for making the determined decision to release the memories, even though they may be the foundation for emotional tears that fall like rain, a heavy rain, even a downpour.

And, even that's okay – the downpouring of tears, that is. Without doubt, the release of all the hurt and shame bottled up inside me is worth every bit of the thunderstorm within my soul when God uses my story to reach out to others who might be hurting, and even to those who might not have ever before had an in-depth understanding of at least *one* who has been a part of the unexpected, *unwed, teenage mother* world.

I gave my testimony in church for the first time ever in October, 2009. Note that this was not only the first time I ever gave my testimony in church, but this was also the first time I ever gave my testimony *anywhere*. As I mentioned very early in this book, this was truly a gargantuan step and leap of faith for me.

I had no idea of how others would react to my story, my unveiling of my *real* self.

To my surprise, my *pleasant* surprise, I had many folks come to me that same day, and even weeks afterward to tell me how much they appreciated my story or how they were moved by my straightforwardness and revealing of myself. Even teenagers came to me, which thrilled me beyond belief, because my heart goes out to each and every one of them in the most genuine way.

It would not surprise me, however, if some of the folks who said nothing at all might be not unlike those same folks who voiced negativities regarding *girls like me* when they didn't know that I *was one of those girls*.

But, I'm even okay with that. After thirty-five years of self-induced embarrassment, it's *finally* ok with me.

For the first time in these thirty-five long years, I can truthfully say, *"It doesn't matter anymore."*

What *does* matter, is that now God can use me.

After all this time, I am finally allowing God to use me for His glory by sharing my story which includes all my shortcomings, my past failures, and my history, as well as my genuine concern and love for especially the teen generation.

What a weight lifted!

Hallelujah!

PART THREE

TAKE A CHANCE ON A TEENAGER

CHAPTER NINE

BEFRIENDING TEENAGERS

*"Let no one despise your youth,
But be an example to believers in word,
In conduct, in love, in spirit, in faith, in purity."
1 Timothy 4: 12*

Is curiosity getting the best of you at this moment, causing you to question why I would regard it crucial to write a chapter concerning the significance of befriending teenagers, especially when the title of this story does not even hint at its inclusion?

Perhaps then, a revisitation of chapters two, three, and four is in order. The teenager's life, as we who have *been there* know all too well, is not an easy road.

And, it is my belief that we who have *been there* have a responsibility to assist present-day teenagers in maneuvering the potholes found all too often on Adolescent Road.

More than likely, you share the hope that I do – that our futures are bright and protected, let alone deemed valuable, especially as we approach older adulthood.

Consider this, folks. Teenagers *are* a whopping big part of our future. If we don't befriend them *now* and take care of their needs, physical as well as emotional, how then can we expect them to have any interest in lending a supportive hand when *we* are elderly or disabled and may require *their* assistance?

I do recognize that teenagers can be difficult at times. But - newsflash! … Just as recognizable, if not more so at times, is the certainty that adults possess equivalent thorny capacities, including *yours truly*.

Not too infrequently, I have aggravated even myself with my own occasional outlandish behaviors, my view of what's *really* important or what *really* matters having been obstructed by my own selfish desires.

And, if I am capable of being an annoyance to even myself periodically, how much more so must I be a real pain to others during those times?

The bottom line is that we all have our *bad* days. We all have those days when we're *just not quite ourselves*. Or, *are we … ourselves?*

In review – no, all teenagers are *not* alike, though they do share a resemblance to one another in that they are each yearning to find their own purpose, and desiring desperately to just *fit in somewhere* – *anywhere*.

I would suggest to you to seize any and all opportunities to walk side-by-side with teenagers down Adolescent Road, and assist them in identifying the sometimes perilous potholes.

Please note, however, that even though we may show them how to maneuver the hazardous potholes while pointing out the risks and dangers of even taking *just a peek* into those potholes, that's not a guarantee they won't just jump in with both feet anyways.

Some might even *dive* head first, in fact, into the wicked ruts.

But, even at those times when teens seemingly refuse to listen to our reasoning, throwing all caution and good sense to the wind, it's so important that we're there for them, readily available to offer our hand, to pull them out, to lift them up, and to be their support.

I've had plenty of my own *head-first* moments, much to my regret.

On the flip side, it is those same *head-first* moments that serve as the driving force in causing me to make at least a small portion of my life story an *open book*, rather than keeping my skeleton's mouth clamped tightly shut.

My dear mom and dad offered their precious hands, pulling me from plenty of potholes – some much deeper than others – and many more than I will mention in the pages of this particular story.

Sure, there were those instances when my naïve, teenage mind questioned whether I wanted to grab my parents' helping hands immediately as opposed to waiting awhile; as well as those times when I wasn't quite certain if I even wanted to grab hold of their devoted hands at all.

But, there were quite a number of times when I readily offered my scared-stiff, outstretched arms in acceptance of their merciful hands, and grabbed hold with the tightest of grips.

What would I have done without their unconditionally loving support?

I shudder to think of the direction my life might have taken without their guidance … especially, *post*-potholes.

I cannot imagine that there is any *loving* parent who would have a preference for the *"learning by experience"* method in order for their own children to realize the dangers of life's potholes.

Sadly however, history has shown us too clearly and too often that there have been countless parents who were not quite so loving, exhibiting no evidence of regard for the positive nurture of their own children. My heart goes out to these *"kids"*, whoever they are and whatever their age. I pray for them as well as their parents.

If, per chance, you are a parent whose child has chosen to jump or dive into a risky pothole, and maybe even continues to sink deeper with each passing day – know this: there is a way out.

Sometimes though, the *way out* may take a little longer for your child as compared with someone else's child. Or, the *route* your child takes in order climb out of the hole may be a distinctively different path than another child may choose.

Love them through it all.

And regrettably, there will be those kids who never seem to *find their way.*

Love them through all of that, too.

Easier said than done, I'm certain.

Nevertheless, never give up hope that your child will learn from his or her mistakes, become skilled at avoiding dangerous potholes, and grow into the kind of adult who could someday make *you* feel very secure grabbing *his or her* helping hand, allowing him or her to lift *you* up and give *you* support.

It's the *circle of life,* right?

A close friend often asks me, *"What's the secret to befriending the teenager?"* My answer is that there is *no* secret, or at least not one that I've found.

Rather, at least for me, it's more of a personal *motivation* to guard teenagers from the insecurities that seem to routinely invade their psyches … insecurities that have the potential of leading their precious, youthful feet directly into the dreaded potholes.

My personal motivation to be the *pothole crossing guard* for teenagers originates from my own regrettable familiarity with the misery that potholes impart to the unsuspecting adolescent; as well as a heartfelt desire to safely lead kids from *teendom* into the *territory of adulthood.*

If you've never experienced *teenage potholes,* or even if your experience with them was minimal, it might take a little more practice for you to earn your *badge* identifying you as a competent *pothole crossing guard.* But they say, *"practice makes perfect."*

And, though teenagers aren't necessarily looking for *perfection*, they just might be looking for at least a smidgen of *practice* on the part of the adult population.

Since I seem to have a built-in personal interest in teenagers, I think *practicing as crossing guard* might just come a little more natural for me. Well, that and the fact that I have *been there*.

Could my sense of ease around teenagers be the result of having missed out on the greater portion of my teenage years, and I'm trying to recapture that part of my childhood?

Could be ... but, I doubt it.

My dad is intrinsically partial to teenagers, as well. Could it be that my soft spot for teenagers was passed from my father's genes to my own?

Could be.

All teenagers are entitled to our attention, acceptance, concern, understanding, and love.

When our own children were growing up, we realized the importance of giving them *D.E.A.L. time* ("*drop everything and listen" time*).

Incontestably though, it's true that hindsight is 20/20.

That being said, it sure would be nice to be able to go back in time, being considerably more aware of how very precious the *D.E.A.L.* moments with our children really were, and allowing even more – much more – cherished time for those moments.

We *all* like to be heard, *especially* while we're teenagers, when ...

- Our hormones are running *amuck*.
- But, we're not even certain what hormones are.
- We're told we *shouldn't* act like *children*.
- We're told we *can't* be treated as adults.
- We don't think our *parents* understand us at all.
- We don't think our *teachers* understand us at all.

- We're not even totally convinced our *friends* understand us.
- We *want* to be like everyone else.
- We *don't want* to be like everyone else.
- We need our *friends*.
- But, we need our *space* too.
- We need a lot of sleep.
- But, we don't want to sleep. (Or, we don't want to follow the same sleep schedule as the rest of the world.)
- We *think* we know-it-all.
- So, we share our *brainpower* with those whom we deem of significantly lower intelligence; e.g., our parents.
- But, our parents quickly *put us in our place*.

Which brings us *full circle* to the *confusion vs. confidence* point I made earlier in this text.

It's no secret that teenagers have a strong desire to be confident, but there's so much confusing riff raff coming at them like ants at a picnic that it's no wonder teenagers are confused, let alone *stressed* (even though it goes against all the unwritten rules of the adolescent world for them to admit to any inkling of such nervous tension).

Methods I've personally discovered to be effective in assisting teenagers to *de-stress* follow.

- Relax!
- *You* make the first move in initiating conversation.
- If *they* make the first move, respond as if you have all the time in the world. (Do you *really* have something so terribly important to attend to that you can't *make time* and *take time?*)
- *Really* listen to what they're saying to you.
- Then, make a genuine effort to *remember* what they said to you, and continue with the same topic the next time

you see them. (They're not dim-witted. They'll know if your initial interest in them was counterfeit.)

- Look the teenager in the eyes, and with a heartfelt smile.
- Give them a hug when you see them.
- Give them a hug when you leave them.
- Know who their friends are.
- Befriend their friends.
- If it's not your child, be friends with their parents.
- Find the *good* in them, and compliment them on it … over and over again.
- If you find something *not-so-good* in them, pray about it, and ask them about it when the *timing* is appropriate. (*Timing* is more important than you might think.) If the teen is *your own child,* sooner is better than later. If the teen is *someone else's child,* it's *not* your place to scold or lecture, but you *can* gently point them in a better direction.
- Do *something* with them that interests them.
- Do *nothing* with them, because sometimes they like to just sit and do *nothing in particular.*
- Laugh with them.
- Cry with them.
- Be silly with them.
- Tell them some of the silly stuff you did as a teenager.
- Find a mutual interest, and build on your friendship by *sharing* that interest.

RELAXING

Take a good look around the next time you are in *mixed company* – the company that includes teenagers as well as adults. Too often, there is a sensation of edginess that appears to hover in the air like a dark cloud.

This especially bowls me over since in order to reach adulthood, we were **all** required first to maneuver the potholes of adolescence.

Perhaps some folks just exit one uneasy stage of life only to find themselves stepping straight into yet another tense amphitheater, except that on this particular *stage*, it is not only a prerequisite that we have been on the stage of adolescence, but also that we were *supposed* to have gathered a substantial amount of maturity at least somewhere along the way.

Maybe if more of us would make a conscious and determined effort to loosen up around teenagers by approaching them with a deliberate mindset to form a friendly relationship, the uneasiness would disappear, thus allowing relaxation to make itself more *at home,* and even settle in for the long haul.

MAKING THE FIRST MOVE

It's important to have a learned awareness of when it *is* and when it *isn't* appropriate to make the first move toward friendships with teenagers. There's a fine line to be monitored there; and it must never, ever be crossed.

But, don't let that *fine line* scare you. It is my belief that there is nothing wrong with approaching the *fine line* as long as you keep a dignified and respectable distance, while at the same time acknowledging to the teenager that he or she really *is somebody* and that he or she has an important role to play in this sometimes confusing world.

BEING THERE WHEN THEY MAKE THE FIRST MOVE

There's not really a certain type of teenager who will always make the *first move*. It does not matter whether they are outgoing or shy, smart or not-so-smart, popular or unpopular. Teens from all walks of life and personality types have been known to make that *first move.*

My experience has been that when a teen *does* make that first move, it is usually because you have said something or done something that has shown them that you are *real, genuine, human,* and *accepting.*

So, when they make that first move, whether it's just a simple *"hello"*, a smile, or an initiation of conversation – keep it going. Smile. Say *"hello"* back, and keep talking. Let *them* be the ones to end the conversation. Not you!

LISTENING

Whatever you do, don't *pretend* you're listening. Really listen. If you fake it, the teenager will uncover the truth probably sooner rather than later, and then you'll really have to work long and hard toward recovering the lost trust, let alone the friendship.

REMEMBERING WHAT THEY SAID

Don't be mistaken. There *will* be a test.

Yes, the teen will test you at a later date(s) to determine not only whether or not you were truly listening when he or she was talking, but also to determine whether or not you had any genuine interest at all in his or her remarks.

If the making of *mental* notes is not an option for you, make *pen and paper* notes.

Don't worry about whether or not someone happens to come across your notes. If they do happen upon them, it'll just make for conclusive evidence of your genuine interest.

I'm reasonably good at making *mental* notes myself, but I'm not at all against making the *pen and paper* kind, if I reach the point where my memory is *not what it used to be*. Trust me – it's definitely reaching that point.

Wait!

What memory?

Yeah, I acquired *that gene* from my dad, too. He has always kept a miniature notebook with him specifically to purposefully jot down information that is worthy of remembering regarding different folks he encounters, whatever their age. It has served him well for many years – well, at least for as long as I can remember.

SMILING

Don't be a cliché'. Don't be a *grumpy old man* or a *crabby old lady*. And, yes – if you are not a teenager yourself, you are most definitely *old* to the teenager. In fact, everybody from about the age of 25 through 105 is *old* in the mind of the teenager.

Don't kid yourself about this very important fact. You're young only once. And if you're not under the age of twenty-five, you're not so young anymore, at least not to the teenager.

As a matter of fact, to the teenager everybody from 25 to 105 stands under the same *uni-age* umbrella, or at least within a short walking distance from each other, but *miles upon miles* from that youthful teen umbrella. It doesn't make any difference how *young-at-heart* you might feel.

HUGGING THEM

Is it acceptable for an adult to *hug* a teenager?

My opinion is this: As long as the hug is one that serves *only* to let the teenager know that his or her existence is one that matters; and that the hug does *not* give anyone – *anyone at all* – the impression that the hug was meant for anything more than that … then, by all means – yes! Of course, it's okay.

Additionally, I feel duty-bound to add that any such physical display of affection **must** be carried out with tremendous discernment; and ought *only* to be shown *in the presence of other respectable adults* who know you very well and are extremely familiar with the simple, genuine, and *blameless intents* of your heart.

BEING FRIENDS WITH THEIR FRIENDS

Their *friends* can be your greatest resource. Observe closely. You should be able to discern what common ground the teen has with his or her friends.

It'll give you something to talk about the next time you encounter the teen ... especially when the teen approaches you with just a smile or a simple *"hello"*, and then just stands there waiting patiently for *you* to be the one that keeps that conversation going.

BEING FRIENDS WITH THEIR PARENTS

Their *parents* can be your greatest resource. Oh, wait! Didn't I just say that about their friends?

The bottom line is that *both* friends *and* parents of teenagers are great resources for forming life-long bonds with teenagers.

Don't just observe this time, though.

Really get to know them. Invite them over.

Make sure the parents understand your intentions, and recognize that you are not a threat to their own positive relationship with their child.

REACTING TO THE GOOD IN THEM

They do, too, have *good* in them!

In fact, they were born with it. Though they might have temporarily misplaced the *good,* it's still there – somewhere amongst all the dirt from the potholes they wandered into. You might just have to *dig* through all the grime in order to find it.

Treat it like a *treasure hunt.* And when you find it, cherish every blessed minute of it. That way it'll be easier to continue to love them when you come across the *not-so-good* characteristics.

REACTING TO THE NOT-SO-GOOD IN THEM

I am certain it comes as no surprise that they embody some *not-so-good* features, as well. They were born with that, too.

So, what does that make them?

It makes them *no different than anyone else.* We're all born with a *sinful nature.* The Bible tells us so.

D.E.A.L. with it! (Drop everything and listen.)

Likewise, in the card game of life, it's a requirement that they take their turn playing the part of the *DEALer,* as well.

The difference is that when they *"do time"* as DEALer, their *time* ought to be a significantly longer *sentence* when compared with your own *time*.

Specifically here – I am speaking as <u>one parent to another</u>, because in the majority of situations, it is the *parent* who will be (or should be) doing the *sentencing.*

Don't be afraid to let them know the *"L"* in dealing stands for the *listening* part of their *sentence,* as a resulting outcome for their period of *not-so-goodness.*

The hope, of course, is that they'll *listen* <u>and</u> *learn.*

DOING SOMETHING

Don't just sit there – do something.

I've never personally met a teenager who didn't have any interests at all. They've all been interested in at least one thing or another.

Uncover what interests them. Even if it's not something that's of particular interest to you, *ask* them about it.

They like to talk about themselves.

Remember? We *all* like to be heard.

Who knows? It may happen to be something that you're at least interested in hearing and learning more about, if not something that you may consider pursuing yourself.

DOING NOTHING

If you do nothing, that's exactly what you'll get in return – nothing, unless you're doing nothing *with* them.

Pregnant at 16

For instance, let's consider those times when you accuse your children or any other teenager of doing nothing or, *wasting time*.

"Waste it" *with* them.

My experience has been that when I have purposefully done *nothing* with teenagers – whether my own children, or someone else's children – *nothing* turns rather quickly into *something*, which translates into time not wasted.

LAUGHING, CRYING, AND SILLINESS

Don't hide your emotions.

Too often, teenagers already fear we older folks have somewhere along the transition from adolescence to adulthood, morphed into emotionless zombies.

Is it any wonder they're not longing for the day when they become *one of us?* They don't want any part of *that excitement (sarcasm)*.

Go out on a *youthful* limb; cast off your *humdrum* adult hang-ups; let your *lackluster* hair down; take it nice 'n easy; loosen up the monotony; and get into the exhilarating swing of renewing your *young-at-heart* frame of mind.

At least for a while – and surely, while interacting with teenagers.

BUILDING FRIENDSHIPS BASED ON MUTUAL INTERESTS

Review the above points, and try 'em out. And, remember that *"practice makes perfect."*

Subsequently, you should find that the *friendship-building* will fascinatingly emerge as if you've magically pulled that rabbit right out of the teenager's hat.

When you come right down to it, building friendships with teenagers is not too much unlike building friendships while in the company of folks around your own age, except that the adolescent has not had the *years of life experiences* and opportunities for *lessons-*

learned as compared with what you have stumbled upon … *pre* and *post* potholes.

While you're *putting into practice* your friendship-building skills with these soul-searching youths, bear in mind that they are approaching adulthood in *the blink of an eye.*

Think about it. The duration of their journey through adolescence is only eight years. Only eight!

What have *you* accomplished in the last eight years? Probably the same thing *most* adults have accomplished in the same time frame.

You got eight years older.

Comparatively then, the *accomplished* adolescent may very well have *accomplished* more than you have in the same period of time. Pretty impressive, I'd say!

Hey, *there's* at least *something* you have in common you've both traveled Adolescent Road.

In view of that common ground, think back to when you were a teenager. Recapture your feelings about *"stuff"*, for example:

- The way you saw the world.
- What you truly believed would make the world a better place.
- The manner in which you wanted to be treated by everyone.
- The manner in which you desired to be talked to by adults.
- The manner in which you yearned to be heard by adults.

Furthermore, don't make the mistake of interacting with teenagers in a manner that is always about maturing. Teenagers already feel like they're going to be stuck in that *maturing classroom* for *forever-and-a-day.*

Make it light and enjoyable. Don't always go into *"parenting mode."*

Good grief! Don't they get enough of that at home? Do they have to get it from you, too?

I promise, that'll be their *train of thought* if you choose to continuously turn on the *parent-attitude*. 'Cause if you buy a ticket for *that train ride*, it won't make a *hill-of-beans* difference if you thought you bought a one-way ticket to teen-land.

Nope. The ticket you unwittingly procured will most assuredly become *not* one-way, but round-trip. Destination: Nowhere. Right back where you started.

CHAPTER 10
BEFRIENDING PREGNANT TEENAGERS

*"A new commandment I give to you,
That you love one another;
As I have loved you, that you also love one another."
John 13: 34*

How do you go about befriending – let alone, loving - the *unwed, pregnant* teenager?

I would suggest following my mom's example. It's the *best* illustration that I know of, personally.

Yeah, I know. You're probably thinking, *"Of course she loved you, you goofball – she's your mother."*

You're right. She *is* my mother. But, I'm no goofball.

I recognize a good friend when I see one. And, she is a true friend if ever I saw one. She is:

- Loving
- Fun
- Attentive
- Supportive
- Caring

- Honest
- Trustworthy
- Accepting
- Loyal
- Dependable
- Patient
- Understanding
- Emotionally Uplifting

And, most importantly …

- Always there for me. *Always!*

Remember? I already mentioned in a previous chapter that she is my peer. I am in her peer group. And I'm proud of it, and proud of her.

When I was a pregnant teenager, she didn't *have* to be my friend. It wasn't a requirement. She could've just remained in mother-mode. And when the time came, grandmother-mode.

But, she chose *not* to *stay put* in any particular mode. Rather, she *was* and *still is* everything to me.

She's *always* gone that extra mile.

And, when I consider the heartrending miles she must have walked in her precious shoes during 1974, while I was pregnant with Danny, I am speechless – lost in the tear-jerking reflections of how seemingly tirelessly she worked to make *me* feel cherished. Me!

All the attributes held by my mother during my teen pregnancy, continue to be held by her today.

All the attributes my mother continues to hold, are the attributes needed to befriend the unwed, pregnant teenage girl.

The only difference, though quite a significant one, between the unwed, pregnant teenager and any other teenager is that she's a little more confused, a little more frightened, and much more concerned about friendships and being accepted by others.

Additionally, if she's decided to keep her baby, she's incontestably concerned about her ability to be a good mother.

If she's decided to put her baby up for adoption, more than likely she's concerned that her baby will be raised in a loving home, by loving parents, and given opportunities that she may have missed out on for one reason or another.

If she's decided to have an abortion, I *plead* with you to do all you can do to help her understand that there are <u>other options</u>.

I stress this point, because so often young, unwed, teenage girls don't recognize that the unexpected pregnancy is *not the end* of the world … that it is *not the end* of all things good and wonderful … that it is *not the end* of their youth … and, that it is *not the end* of their being lovingly accepted by others.

But, these teenage girls also very often do not realize that their decision for abortion *IS the ending* of a precious life.

Do all you can to help this young lady be *informed*. If you feel you don't have the expertise needed in that area – for goodness sake, point her in the direction of someone who *is* an expert.

If you don't personally know an expert, look it up in your phone book – being confident that you are locating telephone numbers of agencies that are pro-life; e.g., *pregnancy care centers* whose business it is to protect the lives of the unborn, as well as to lovingly educate the mom-to-be.

Whatever you do, don't just sit there, doing nothing. Don't allow yourself to become complacent on the abortion issue. And, don't allow yourself to merely *sit back and wait to see what happens*.

Sitting back and waiting to see what happens is shameful, especially for the born-again Christian.

Do something, anything, no matter how small you think your *something* is.

Whatever your *something* may be, you might just discover that it was a very *BIG* something in the eyes of an unwed, pregnant teenager.

PART FOUR

GODS BLESSING

CHAPTER ELEVEN
BLESSINGS BEYOND MY DREAMS

"Likewise you younger people, submit yourselves to your elders.
Yes, all of you be submissive to one another,
And be clothed with humility,
For God resists the proud but gives grace to the humble.
Therefore, humble yourselves under the mighty hand of God,
That He may exalt you in due time,
Casting all your care upon Him, for He cares for you.
Be sober, be vigilant;
Because your adversary the devil walks about like a roaring lion,
Seeking whom he may devour.
Resist him, steadfast in the faith,
Knowing that the same sufferings
Are experienced by your brotherhood in the world."
1 Peter 5: 5-9

My teen pregnancy and the birth of Danny made me grow up fast.

Yes, my own personal *teen-aging process* passed by much more quickly than I had originally anticipated early on in my travels down Adolescent Road.

In fact, I actually *passed by* rather a great deal of the whole teenage process, rather than muddling *through* its entirety.

Nonetheless, my pregnancy and Danny's subsequent presence in my life pushed me full force into the world of adulthood and consequently, made me a little more mature. Although some of my close friends might deny the *maturity* part due to my present-day, occasionally mischievous *"schemes"*.

Undoubtedly, these friends are probably thinking, *"A little more mature? Put the emphasis on 'little'."*

And if, indeed, that *is* what they're thinking, it's okay, simply because my closest friends know me *that well*, and know that I'm *admittedly* a fan of the saying, *"Growing old is mandatory. Growing up is optional."*

But in the grand *"scheme"* of things, and in the course of my everyday life since I was an unwed, pregnant, sixteen year old girl in 1974, I can finally say that I am contentedly satisfied with whom I have become.

More importantly, I am thankful for God's mercy and grace for transforming my seemingly hopeless, teenage situation into – as my high school teacher once said – a *"blessing beyond my dreams."*

As a portion of the Scripture reference at the beginning of this chapter refers to, I did *"cast all my care upon Him"*. And, the Lord helped me to *"resist the devil"*, and significantly raised my consciousness that the devil is constantly walking about *"like a roaring lion, seeking whom he may devour."*

Satan, in fact, works quite determinedly to convince women of all child-bearing ages that abortion is the way to go if a pregnancy is unwanted for whatever reason.

It distresses me immensely that the devil has been outright successful in his devouring these young mothers' minds, especially since 1973 – when abortion became a legalized crime - causing folks to accept the wretchedly false belief that ending a life is superior to giving birth.

I am, in fact, resolutely convinced that there is not one – *NO, NOT ONE* – young, unwed, teenage girl out there who cannot get assistance somewhere/somehow in order to carry her unborn baby to full term; at which time she may either choose to keep the baby, or if need be (for *whatever* reason), choose to give the baby to a loving adoptive family or family member.

From the very depths of my soul, due to not just my own unwed pregnancy experience, but my familiarity with others' experiences as well, and for the reasons listed in the Bible references submitted at the beginning of this book, I believe sex should be saved until marriage.

Hey! That would certainly solve the whole unwed pregnancy issue, wouldn't it?

Think about it! Our common sense even tells the tale of the positive aspects regarding saving sex until marriage, if not only because when a pregnancy occurs within the bond of marriage, the likelihood of considering abortion is almost non-existent – at least in most cases.

But even then, I am far from naive. I am powerfully aware that since abortion has become a legalized crime, even those who are married may choose death over life in the case of an unexpected pregnancy.

But, *"Be not deceived: God cannot be mocked. A man reaps what he sows. The one who sows to please his sinful nature (or, his flesh), from that nature will reap destruction; the one who sows to please the Spirit (God), from the Spirit will reap eternal life." - Galatians 6: 7-8*

I am keenly aware however, that not everyone holds my same pro-life views; let alone my views regarding the institution of marriage, as well as the importance of being a believer in Christ.

That being the case, if you are unable or unwilling to control your sexual drives, at least control your mind as it relates to good vs. evil, life vs. death, and birth vs. abortion.

We've come a long way from the *stone age*. Use protection!

If a pregnancy occurs despite the protection, it does not bring the *responsible* parties' *responsibilities* to a halt. In spite of everything, the unborn child is silently resting in the expectation that his or her momma will not resort to drastic measures.

Those of us who passionately oppose abortion have been and continue to be relentlessly criticized by our opponents because we are the voice for the unborn children who have no voice, let alone no choice in the matter.

The criticism is particularly persistent when we announce to those on the *other side* that our minds are especially boggled that they would dub their proponents *pro-choice*.

Are you kidding me?

Call a spade a spade.

My side promotes ourselves as pro-life, because we believe in the sanctity of life. We are *for* life.

Yet, their side, which holds the extreme opposite view of the pro-lifers, has the audacity – no, cowardice - to promote themselves as pro-choice, when in fact they are pro-death.

Yes, they are!

It doesn't at all boggle my *own* pro-life mind that those who are pro-death, call themselves pro-choice. Pro-choice just sounds a whole lot less gruesome, doesn't it?

Where's *their* truth-in-advertising?

Wait! I know where *their truth* went. Out the window!

There's <u>no</u> *gray area* in this debate.

As for me, my own teenage reckless sexual behaviors resulted in a pregnancy. But not once – <u>NOT ONCE!</u> – have I regretted my decision to choose life for Danny.

And, Danny has certainly exceeded my expectations by providing me with *blessings beyond my dreams.* If I didn't choose life for Danny, for instance, I wouldn't have been blessed with:

- The joy beyond measure that only a son can bring.
- Seeing the pride in Danny's eyes when he caught his first fish.

- The thrill of announcing, *"That's _my_ son"*, as Danny received his trophy for coming in first place at the Pinewood Derby.
- Frogs for pets.
- Danny's eight year old voice proclaiming, *"I'm the happiest boy in the world"*, while on the kitchen floor playing with his brand new puppy, Copper.
- Watching Danny grab his fishing pole after school, and sit for hours fishing off the bridge that ran across the creek in the back yard of our home.
- The pleasure of watching Danny get baptized at the pond across the street from the small, country church we attended.
- A son who repeatedly demonstrates how to be friends with everybody.
- A lovely daughter-in-law.
- And, the joy-beyond-measure of my first grandchild, Lindsey.

My high school teacher was right.

God really has blessed me beyond my dreams!

AFTERWORD

*"Fear not, for I am with you.
Be not dismayed for I am your God.
I will strengthen you,
Yes, I will help you.
I will uphold you with my righteous right hand."
Isaiah 41: 10*

Have I detailed *all* the skeletons in my closet? No. I still have a few.

But, sometimes it's best to keep some things a mystery.

Yes, it is!

After having read this book in its entirety, you might be wondering, *"By what authority has Lori been given the right to author such a book as this?"*

Though my experiences may not have made me an *expert* by your standards, they have indeed at least made me a *specialist* of sorts, in the same manner that many of your own experiences have given you authorization to speak out and make your *own* voice heard.

After all, *experience* is a teacher of sorts, right?

You know the saying, *"Your child holds your hand for a little while, but holds your heart forever?"* Let me additionally suggest this to you … Never, ever let go of your child's heart and make certain *your* hands are always lovingly accessible.

Yes, that's another one of those *lessons learned* from my own parents over the years.

That's not to advocate leading your child around by the nose until the day you die.

Without doubt, it's important that we teach our children how to make it on their own and to guide them in such a way that they become responsible adults.

But it is my conviction that, even more importantly and unquestionably, parents ought to let their children of whatever age know that their hands and even their arms are ever-present and always available for emotional support.

Many thanks are extended to all my family and friends, from the bottom of my heart, for doing so much more than just *"being there"*.

I love you.

A final thought for my readers to ponder:

How can we expect the frightened, confused, unwed, pregnant teenager to make the very right decision for life when she is relentlessly attacked by shameful fingers and fiery darts?